The
Complete
DASH DIET
Cookbook for Beginners

2000 Days Quick & Easy Nutrient-Rich Recipes to Manage Blood Pressure Naturally

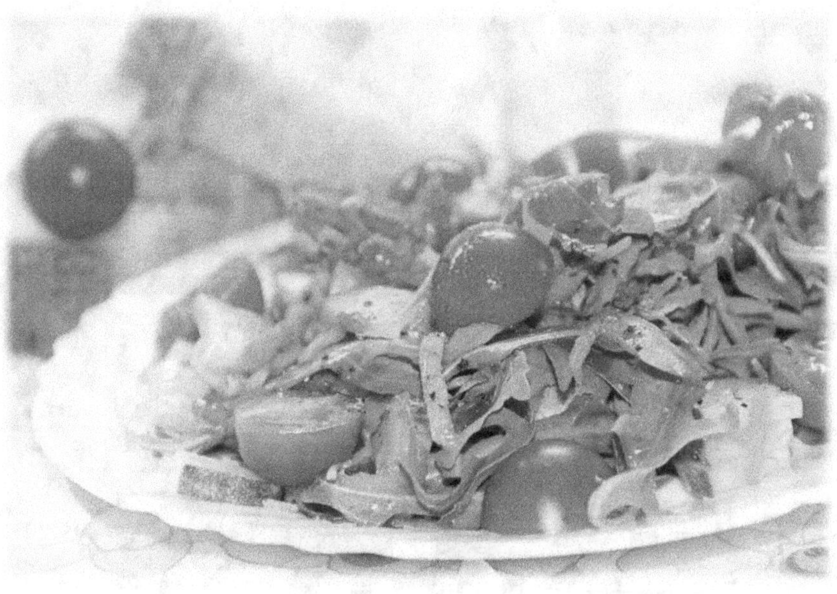

Eric A. Randell

ERIC A. RANDELL

COPYRIGHT

SCAN HERE FOR MORE BOOKS FROM ME

TABLE OF CONTENTS

INTRODUCTION

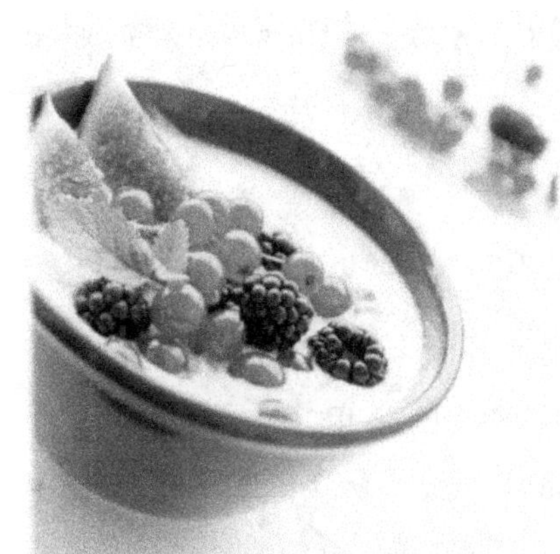

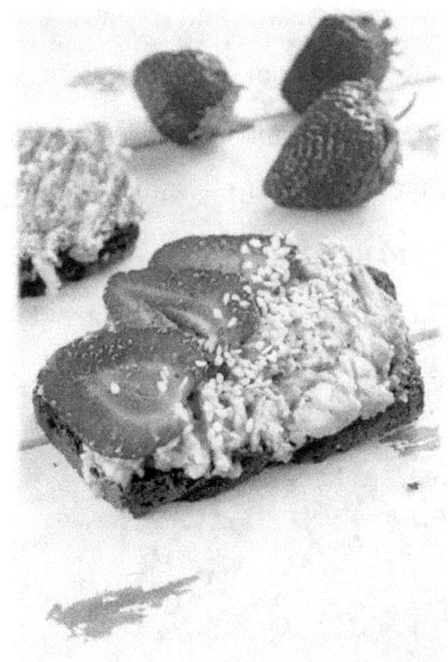

Are you tired of fad diets that promise the world but never deliver? Do you struggle with high blood pressure and wonder if there's a way to manage it through nutrition? Look no further, because the Dash Diet Cookbook for Beginners is here to change the way you think about healthy eating.

In a world filled with processed foods and quick-fix diets, it's easy to lose sight of the importance of a balanced diet. But the truth is, what you put into your body has a direct impact on your overall health and well-being. And for those struggling with high blood pressure, the right diet can make all the difference.

The Dash Diet, which stands for Dietary Approaches to Stop Hypertension, is a scientifically proven way to lower blood pressure and improve overall heart health. By focusing on fruits, vegetables, lean proteins, and whole grains, the Dash Diet offers a sustainable and effective way to manage high blood pressure without relying on medication alone.

In this cookbook, you'll find a collection of delicious and easy-to-make recipes that are specifically designed for beginners. From hearty salads to flavorful stir-fries, each recipe is thoughtfully crafted to help you transition to a healthier way of eating without feeling deprived or overwhelmed.

So, if you're ready to take control of your health and explore the power of a balanced diet, the Dash Diet Cookbook for Beginners is your ultimate guide. Say goodbye to restrictive and unrealistic diets, and say hello to a sustainable and enjoyable way of eating that will leave you feeling your best. Say hello to the Dash Diet.

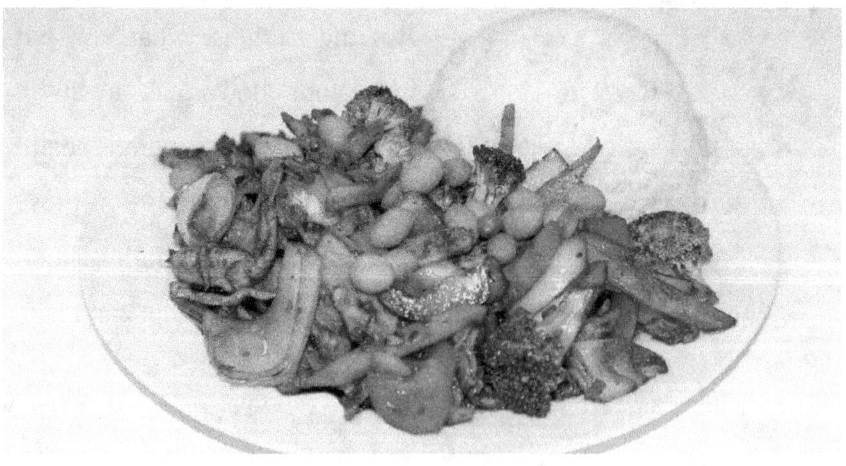

UNDERSTANDING DASH DIETS AND ITS IMPORTANCE

The DASH diet, which stands for Dietary Approaches to Stop Hypertension, is a dietary plan specifically designed to help lower high blood pressure. It emphasizes consuming foods rich in nutrients like potassium, calcium, protein, and fiber, as well as reducing sodium intake. The DASH diet is recognized as an effective and sustainable way to manage high blood pressure without the sole reliance on medication.

For individuals with hypertension, following the DASH diet is particularly important due to its potential to significantly impact blood pressure levels. High blood pressure, or hypertension, is one of the major risk factors for heart disease, stroke, and other serious health-related conditions. By focusing on whole, natural foods and reducing the intake of processed and high-sodium foods, the DASH diet can help lower blood pressure and therefore reduce the risk of developing these cardiovascular diseases.

One of the key reasons DASH diets are important for patients with hypertension is their ability to effectively manage blood pressure levels. The emphasis on fruits, vegetables, whole grains, lean proteins, and low-fat dairy products, combined with limiting highly processed foods, can result in lower blood pressure levels within a relatively short period.

Additionally, the DASH diet is not only beneficial for lowering blood pressure, but it also promotes overall heart health. The nutrient-rich foods recommended by the DASH diet can contribute to reduced cholesterol levels and improved cardiovascular function. This can help prevent further complications related to high blood pressure and reduce the likelihood of heart-related illnesses.

The DASH diet is crucial for patients with hypertension because it provides a well-balanced, sustainable approach to managing blood pressure and promoting heart health. Its focus on nutrient-dense foods and reduction of sodium intake make it a valuable tool in preventing and managing high blood pressure, and ultimately reducing the risk of heart disease and related complications.

RECOMMENDED FOODS FOR HYPERTENSION PATIENTS

1. Fruits: A variety of fruits, including potassium and fiber-rich options like berries, citrus fruits, apples, and bananas.

2. Vegetables: Incorporate diverse vegetables, particularly leafy greens (e.g., spinach, and kale) and cruciferous vegetables (e.g., broccoli, Brussels sprouts).

3. Whole Grains: Opt for whole grain products such as brown rice, quinoa, oatmeal, and whole wheat bread, known for their high fiber content.

4. Lean Proteins: Choose lean protein sources like chicken breast, turkey, fish, tofu, and legumes, which are lower in saturated fat.

5. Low-fat Dairy: Include low-fat or fat-free dairy products like milk, yogurt, and cheese to benefit from their calcium and protein content.

6. Nuts, Seeds, and Legumes: Incorporate heart-healthy fats, protein, and fiber by adding almonds, walnuts, chia seeds, flaxseeds, and various beans and lentils to meals.

7. Healthy Fats: Use sources of healthy fats such as olive oil, avocados, and fatty fish like salmon and mackerel in moderation.

FOODS TO LIMIT FOR HYPERTENSION PATIENTS

1. Sodium: Minimize consumption of high-sodium foods such as processed snacks, canned soups, deli meats, and fast food, as excess sodium can elevate blood pressure.

2. Saturated and Trans Fats: Reduce intake of foods high in saturated and trans fats, including fried foods, fatty meats, and full-fat dairy products, to support heart health.

3. Added Sugars: Decrease consumption of sugary foods and beverages such as soda, candy, pastries, and sweetened cereals, to mitigate potential adverse effects on blood pressure and overall health.

4. Red Meat: Moderate consumption of red and processed meats due to their potential impact on heart health and hypertension.

5. Alcohol: Limit alcohol intake to moderate levels, as excessive consumption can lead to elevated blood pressure.

By following these dietary guidelines, individuals with hypertension can effectively manage their condition and promote overall heart health.

THE ROLE OF EXERCISES AND PHYSICAL ACTIVITIES

Physical activity and exercise play a crucial role in managing high blood pressure and promoting overall cardiovascular health for patients with hypertension. Engaging in regular physical activity has been shown to have numerous positive effects on blood pressure, helping to lower elevated levels and reduce the risk of associated complications.

First and foremost, physical activity can contribute to weight management and overall fitness, which are key factors in managing high blood pressure. Regular exercise can help individuals achieve and maintain a healthy weight, reducing the strain on the heart and blood vessels, which can in turn lower blood pressure levels.

Furthermore, engaging in physical activity has a direct impact on the cardiovascular system. It can improve the efficiency of the heart, enhancing its ability to pump blood and oxygen to the body's tissues. Regular exercise can also increase the flexibility and health of the blood vessels, promoting better circulation and potentially lowering blood pressure.

In addition, physical activity has been linked to stress reduction and improved mental well-being. Stress is known to contribute to high blood pressure, so finding ways to manage stress through activities like exercise can have a positive impact on blood pressure levels.

It's important to note that the type and intensity of exercise will vary depending on an individual's overall health and fitness level. Aerobic exercises such as walking, jogging, swimming, and cycling are often recommended for individuals with high blood pressure, as they can have a significant impact on cardiovascular health. Strength training, flexibility exercises, and balance activities can also contribute to overall physical fitness and well-being.

However, it's essential for individuals with hypertension to consult with their healthcare provider before starting a new exercise program. This is particularly important if there are existing health conditions or concerns, as healthcare professionals can provide guidance on the most suitable and safe exercise regimen.

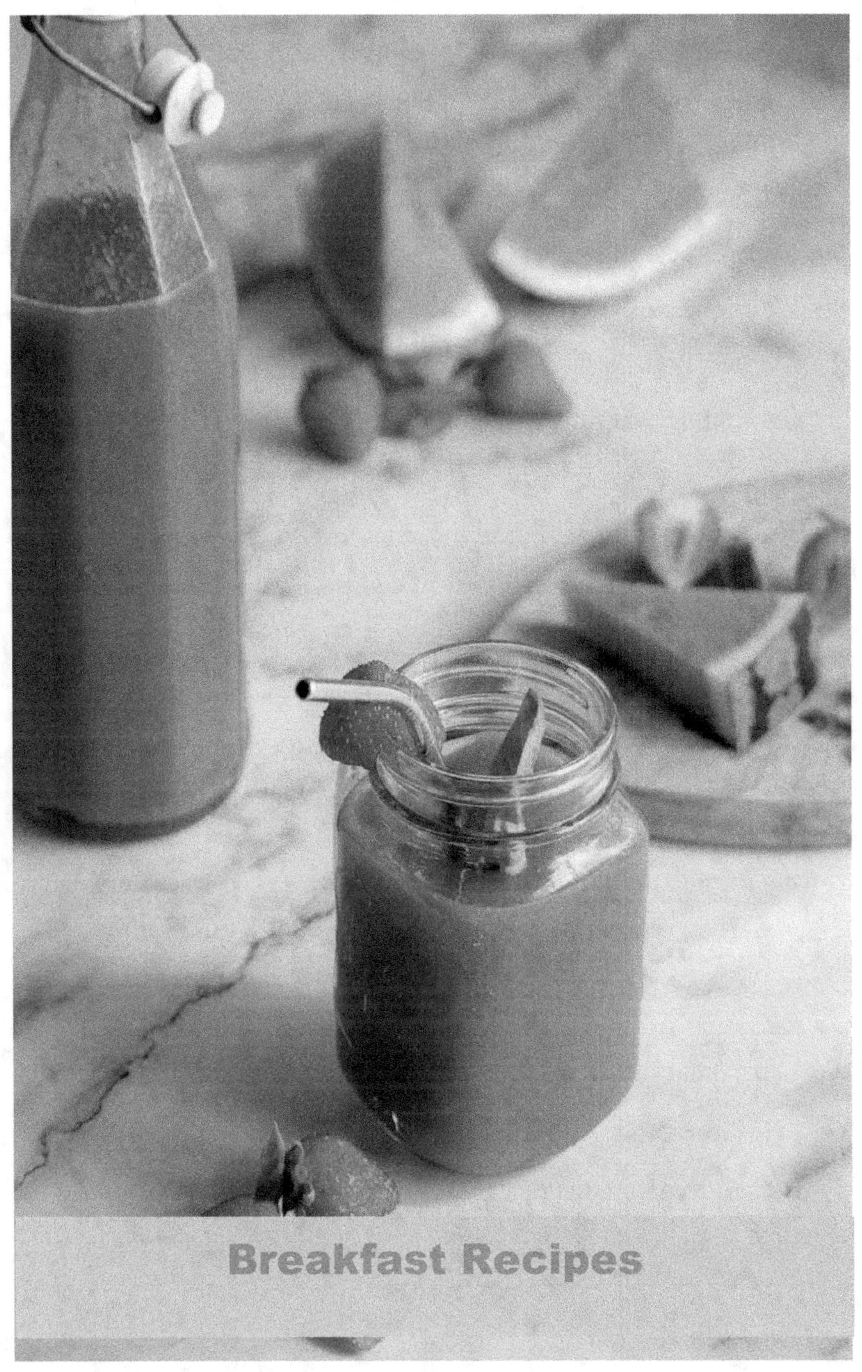
Breakfast Recipes

Greek Yogurt Parfait

Servings: 2 | Prep Time: 10 mins | Cooking Time: 0 mins

Ingredients:

- ❖ 1 cup Greek yogurt
- ❖ 1/2 cup mixed berries
- ❖ 2 tablespoons honey
- ❖ Granola for topping

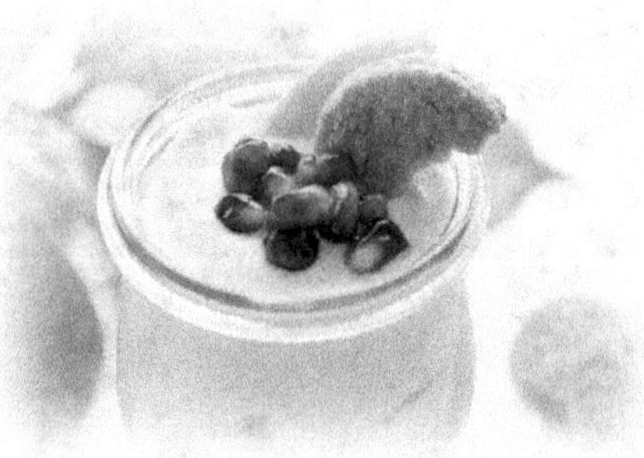

Instructions:

Layer yogurt, berries, and honey in a glass. Top with granola.

Nutritional Info:

Calories: 250, Protein: 15g, Carbs: 40g, Fat: 5g

Avocado Toast

Servings: 2 | Prep Time: 5 mins | Cooking Time: 5 mins

Ingredients:

- ❖ 2 slices whole-grain bread
- ❖ 1 ripe avocado
- ❖ 1 small tomato, sliced
- ❖ Salt and pepper

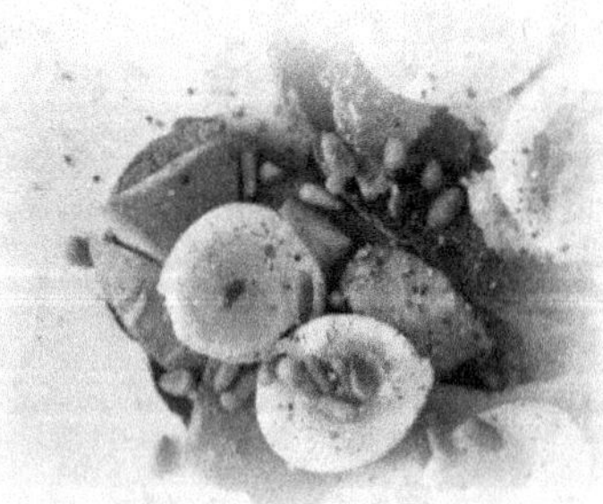

Instructions:

Toast bread, mash avocado on top, add tomato slices, season, and serve.

Nutritional Info:

Calories: 280, Protein: 8g, Carbs: 30g, Fat: 15g

Spinach and Mushroom Omelet

Servings: 2 | Prep Time: 10 mins | Cooking Time: 10 mins

Ingredients:

- ❖ 4 eggs
- ❖ 1 cup spinach
- ❖ 1/2 cup mushrooms, sliced
- ❖ 1/4 cup shredded mozzarella
- ❖ Salt and pepper

Instructions:

Sauté spinach and mushrooms, pour beaten eggs, add cheese, fold, and cook.

Nutritional Info:

Calories: 280, Protein: 20g, Carbs: 4g, Fat: 20g

Banana Nut Oatmeal

Servings: 2 | Prep Time: 5 mins | Cooking Time: 10 mins

Ingredients:

- ❖ 1 cup rolled oats
- ❖ 2 cups almond milk
- ❖ 1 ripe banana, mashed
- ❖ 1/4 cup chopped nuts
- ❖ Cinnamon (optional)

Instructions:

Cook oats in almond milk, stir in banana, top with nuts and cinnamon.

Nutritional Info:

Calories: 320, Protein: 10g, Carbs: 45g, Fat: 12g

Egg and Veggie Breakfast Burrito

Servings: 2 | Prep Time: 10 mins | Cooking Time: 10 mins

Ingredients:

- ❖ 2 whole-grain tortillas
- ❖ 4 eggs, scrambled
- ❖ 1/2 cup bell peppers, diced

- ❖ 1/4 cup onion, chopped
- ❖ 1/4 cup shredded cheddar

Instructions:

Fill tortillas with eggs, veggies, and cheese. Roll and heat on a skillet.

Nutritional Info:

Calories: 330, Protein: 18g, Carbs: 30g, Fat: 15g

Fruit Smoothie Bowl

Servings: 2 | Prep Time: 5 mins | Cooking Time: 0 mins

Ingredients:

- ❖ 2 frozen bananas
- ❖ 1 cup mixed berries
- ❖ 1/2 cup spinach
- ❖ 1/2 cup almond milk
- ❖ Toppings: granola, sliced fruit

Instructions:

Blend bananas, berries, spinach, and almond milk. Pour into bowls, add toppings.

Nutritional Info:

Calories: 240, Protein: 5g, Carbs: 55g, Fat: 3g

Breakfast Quinoa

Servings: 2 | Prep Time: 10 mins | Cooking Time: 5 mins

Ingredients:

- ❖ 1 cup quinoa, cooked
- ❖ 1/2 cup almond milk
- ❖ 1/4 cup chopped nuts
- ❖ 1/4 cup dried fruits (like cranberries)
- ❖ Honey or maple syrup for drizzling

Instructions:

Mix cooked quinoa with almond milk, nuts, fruits, and sweetener. Heat and serve.

Nutritional Info:

Calories: 320, Protein: 10g, Carbs: 50g, Fat: 9g

Cottage Cheese Pancakes

Servings: 2 | Prep Time: 10 mins | Cooking Time: 10 mins

Ingredients:

- ❖ 1 cup cottage cheese
- ❖ 2 eggs
- ❖ 1/4 cup whole wheat flour
- ❖ 1 teaspoon baking powder
- ❖ 1/2 teaspoon vanilla extract

Instructions:

Blend all ingredients, cook batter on a griddle until golden.

Nutritional Info:

Calories: 280, Protein: 25g, Carbs: 20g, Fat: 10g

Breakfast Egg Muffins

Servings: 2 | Prep Time: 10 mins | Cooking Time: 20 mins

Ingredients:

- ❖ 6 eggs
- ❖ 1/2 cup spinach, chopped
- ❖ 1/4 cup bell peppers, diced
- ❖ 1/4 cup diced ham or turkey

❖ Salt and pepper

Instructions:

Whisk eggs, mix in veggies and meat, pour into muffin tin, bake until set.

Nutritional Info:

Calories: 180, Protein: 15g, Carbs: 2g, Fat: 12g

Chia Seed Pudding

Servings: 2 | Prep Time: 5 mins | Chilling Time: 2 hours

Ingredients:

❖ 1/4 cup chia seeds

❖ 1 cup almond milk

❖ 1 tablespoon honey or maple syrup

❖ 1/2 teaspoon vanilla extract

❖ Toppings: sliced fruit, nuts

Instructions:

Mix chia seeds, almond milk, sweetener, and vanilla. Chill, top with fruits and nuts.

Nutritional Info:

Calories: 200, Protein: 6g, Carbs: 20g, Fat: 10g

Blueberry Almond Overnight Oats

Servings: 2 | Prep Time: 5 mins | Cooking Time: 0 mins

Ingredients:

- ❖ 1 cup rolled oats
- ❖ 1 1/2 cups almond milk
- ❖ 1/4 cup blueberries
- ❖ 2 tablespoons almond butter
- ❖ Honey or maple syrup (optional)

Instructions:

Mix oats, almond milk, blueberries, and almond butter. Refrigerate overnight, sweeten if desired.

Nutritional Info:

Calories: 290, Protein: 9g, Carbs: 42g, Fat: 9g

Veggie Breakfast Hash

Servings: 2 | Prep Time: 10 mins | Cooking Time: 20 mins

Ingredients:

- ❖ 2 potatoes, diced
- ❖ 1 bell pepper, diced
- ❖ 1/2 onion, chopped
- ❖ 1 cup spinach
- ❖ 2 eggs
- ❖ Salt, pepper, paprika

Instructions:

Sauté potatoes, bell pepper, and onion until golden. Add spinach, cook until wilted. Fry eggs and serve over hash.

Nutritional Info:

Calories: 320, Protein: 12g, Carbs: 50g, Fat: 8g

Peanut Butter Banana Toast

Servings: 2 | Prep Time: 5 mins | Cooking Time: 5 mins

Ingredients:

- ❖ 2 slices whole-grain bread
- ❖ 2 tablespoons peanut butter

- ❖ 1 banana, sliced
- ❖ Drizzle of honey

Instructions:

Toast bread, spread peanut butter, top with banana slices, and honey.

Nutritional Info:

Calories: 320, Protein: 10g, Carbs: 45g, Fat: 12g

Breakfast Quiche Cups

Servings: 2 | Prep Time: 10 mins | Cooking Time: 20 mins

Ingredients:

- ❖ 4 eggs
- ❖ 1/4 cup milk
- ❖ 1/2 cup spinach, chopped
- ❖ 1/4 cup diced ham
- ❖ 1/4 cup shredded cheddar
- ❖ Salt and pepper

Instructions:

Whisk eggs and milk, add spinach, ham, cheese, salt, and pepper. Pour into muffin tin, bake until set.

Nutritional Info:

Calories: 220, Protein: 15g, Carbs: 4g, Fat: 15g

Apple Cinnamon Quinoa Bowl

Servings: 2 | Prep Time: 5 mins | Cooking Time: 5 mins

Ingredients:

- ❖ 1 cup cooked quinoa
- ❖ 1 apple, diced
- ❖ 1 tablespoon almond butter
- ❖ Cinnamon and nutmeg
- ❖ Almonds for topping

Instructions:

Mix quinoa, apple, almond butter, and spices. Top with almonds.

Nutritional Info:

Calories: 280, Protein: 8g, Carbs: 50g, Fat: 6g

Smoked Salmon Bagel

Servings: 2 | Prep Time: 5 mins | Cooking Time: 5 mins

Ingredients:

- ❖ 2 whole-grain bagels

- ❖ 4 ounces smoked salmon
- ❖ 1/4 cup cream cheese
- ❖ Red onion slices
- ❖ Capers

Instructions:

Toast bagels, spread cream cheese, top with smoked salmon, onion, and capers.

Nutritional Info:

Calories: 350, Protein: 25g, Carbs: 40g, Fat: 12g

Protein-Packed Breakfast Sandwich

Servings: 2 | Prep Time: 10 mins | Cooking Time: 10 mins

Ingredients:

- ❖ 2 whole-grain English muffins
- ❖ 2 eggs
- ❖ 2 slices turkey or chicken bacon
- ❖ 2 slices cheese
- ❖ Spinach leaves

Instructions:

Cook eggs and bacon, assemble on muffins with cheese and spinach.

Nutritional Info:

Calories: 320, Protein: 20g, Carbs: 30g, Fat: 15g

Breakfast Stuffed Peppers

Servings: 2 | Prep Time: 10 mins | Cooking Time: 20 mins

Ingredients:

- ❖ 2 bell peppers, halved
- ❖ 4 eggs
- ❖ 1/2 cup black beans
- ❖ 1/4 cup salsa
- ❖ 1/4 cup shredded cheddar
- ❖ Salt and pepper

Instructions:

Roast peppers, crack eggs into halves, add beans, salsa, cheese, salt, and pepper. Bake until eggs are set.

Nutritional Info:

Calories: 290, Protein: 18g, Carbs: 20g, Fat: 15g

Sweet Potato Breakfast Bowl

Servings: 2 | Prep Time: 10 mins | Cooking Time: 20 mins

Ingredients:

- ❖ 2 cups sweet potatoes, diced
- ❖ 1 tablespoon olive oil
- ❖ 1/4 teaspoon paprika
- ❖ 2 eggs
- ❖ Avocado slices

Instructions:

Roast sweet potatoes with olive oil and paprika. Fry eggs, serve over sweet potatoes with avocado.

Nutritional Info:

Calories: 330, Protein: 10g, Carbs: 40g, Fat: 15g

Tomato Basil Frittata

Servings: 2 | Prep Time: 10 mins | Cooking Time: 20 mins

Ingredients:

- ❖ 6 eggs
- ❖ 1/4 cup milk
- ❖ 1 cup cherry tomatoes, halved

- ❖ 1/4 cup fresh basil, chopped
- ❖ 1/4 cup grated Parmesan
- ❖ Salt and pepper

Instructions:

Whisk eggs and milk, add tomatoes, basil, Parmesan, salt, and pepper. Bake until set.

Nutritional Info:

Calories: 250, Protein: 20g, Carbs: 6g, Fat: 15g

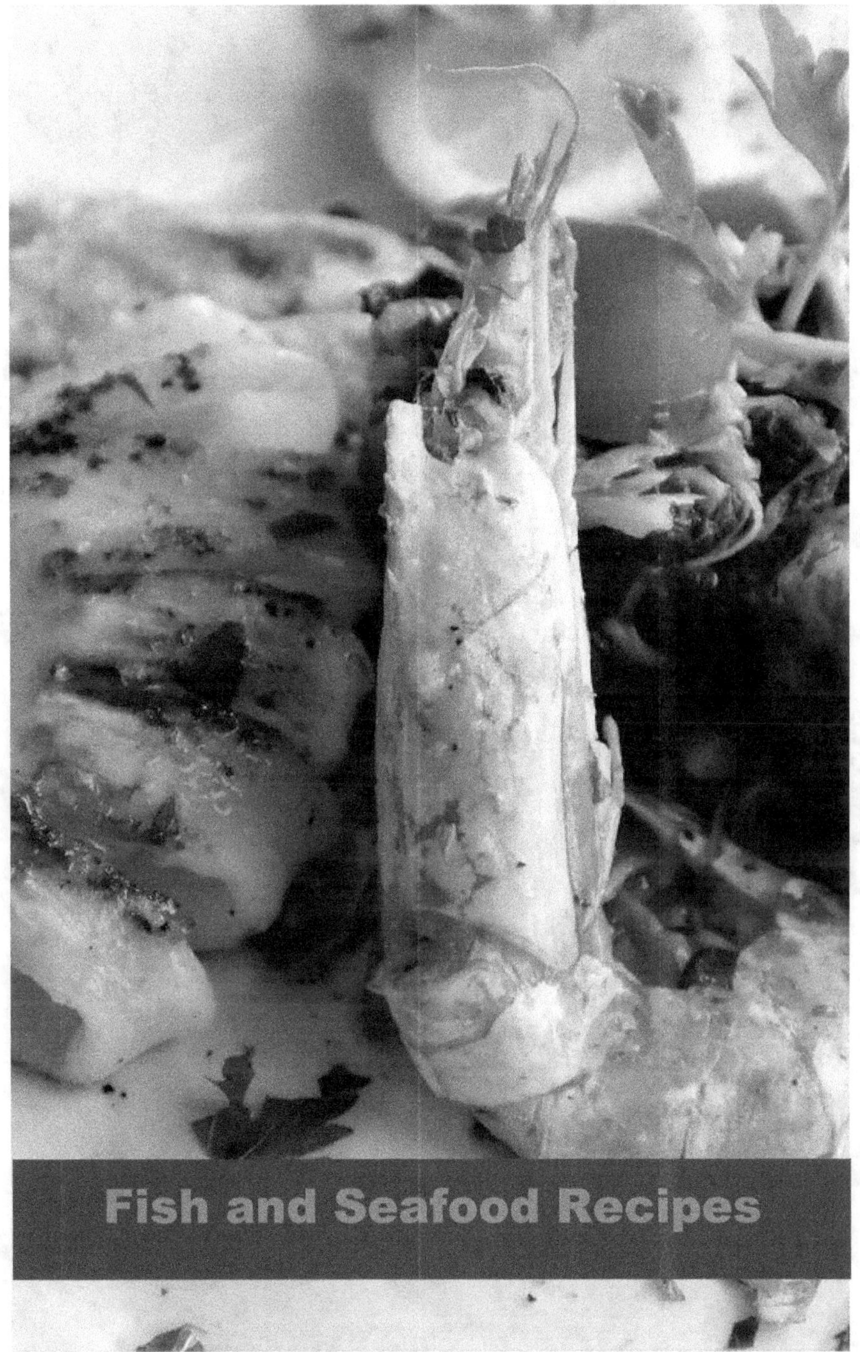
Fish and Seafood Recipes

Lemon Garlic Baked Cod

Servings: 2 | Prep Time: 10 mins | Cooking Time: 15 mins

Ingredients:

❖ 2 cod filets

❖ 2 tablespoons olive oil

❖ 2 cloves garlic, minced

❖ Juice and zest of 1 lemon

❖ Salt, pepper, and parsley

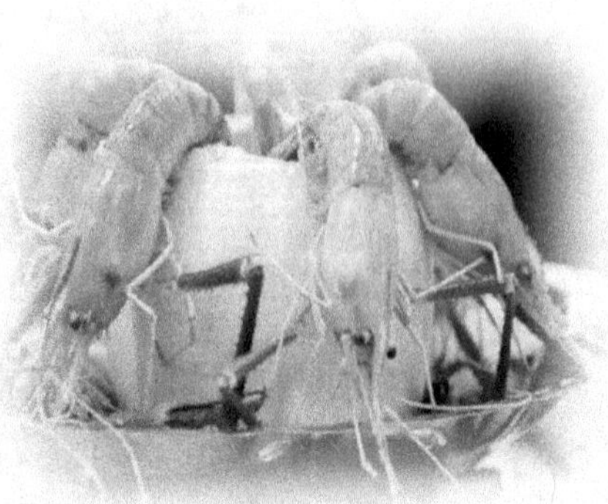

Instructions:

Mix olive oil, garlic, lemon juice, and zest. Marinate cod, bake until fish flakes. Season with salt, pepper, and parsley.

Nutritional Info:

Calories: 200, Protein: 25g, Carbs: 1g, Fat: 10g

Shrimp Stir-Fry

Servings: 2 | Prep Time: 15 mins | Cooking Time: 10 mins

Ingredients:

❖ 1/2-pound shrimp, peeled and deveined

❖ 2 cups mixed vegetables

❖ 2 tablespoons soy sauce

❖ 1 tablespoon sesame oil

❖ 1 clove garlic, minced

❖ Rice or quinoa for serving

Instructions:

Stir-fry shrimp and veggies in sesame oil and garlic. Add soy sauce, cook until shrimp is pink. Serve over rice or quinoa.

Nutritional Info:

Calories: 250, Protein: 25g, Carbs: 15g, Fat: 10g

Grilled Salmon with Dill Sauce

Servings: 2 | Prep Time: 10 mins | Cooking Time: 10 mins

Ingredients:

- 2 salmon filets

- 1 tablespoon olive oil

- Salt, pepper, lemon slices

- Dill Sauce: Greek yogurt, fresh dill, lemon juice

Instructions:

Brush salmon with olive oil, season with salt, pepper, and lemon. Grill until cooked. Serve with dill sauce.

Nutritional Info:

Calories: 300, Protein: 30g, Carbs: 2g, Fat: 18g

Tuna Salad Lettuce Wraps

Servings: 2 | Prep Time: 10 mins | Cooking Time: 0 mins

Ingredients:

- ❖ 1 can tuna, drained
- ❖ 1/4 cup Greek yogurt
- ❖ 1/4 cup diced celery
- ❖ 1/4 cup diced red onion
- ❖ Lettuce leaves for wrapping

Instructions:

Mix tuna, Greek yogurt, celery, and onion. Spoon into lettuce leaves to make wraps.

Nutritional Info:

Calories: 180, Protein: 20g, Carbs: 4g, Fat: 9g

Coconut Shrimp

Servings: 2 | Prep Time: 15 mins | Cooking Time: 15 mins

Ingredients:

- ❖ 1/2-pound shrimp, peeled and deveined
- ❖ 1/2 cup shredded coconut
- ❖ 1/4 cup breadcrumbs
- ❖ 1 egg, beaten
- ❖ Dipping sauce: sweet chili or mango sauce

Instructions:

Dip shrimp in egg, coat with coconut and breadcrumbs. Bake until golden. Serve with dipping sauce.

Nutritional Info:

Calories: 280, Protein: 20g, Carbs: 10g, Fat: 15g

Garlic Butter Scallops

Servings: 2 | Prep Time: 5 mins | Cooking Time: 15 mins

Ingredients:

- ❖ 1/2-pound scallops
- ❖ 2 tablespoons butter
- ❖ 2 cloves garlic, minced
- ❖ Salt, pepper, fresh parsley
- ❖ Lemon wedges for serving

Instructions:

Sear scallops in butter and garlic until golden. Season with salt, pepper, and parsley. Serve with lemon wedges.

Nutritional Info:

Calories: 220, Protein: 25g, Carbs: 2g, Fat: 12g

Baked Halibut with Herb Crust

Servings: 2 | Prep Time: 10 mins | Cooking Time: 15 mins

Ingredients:

- ❖ 2 halibut filets
- ❖ 1/4 cup breadcrumbs
- ❖ 2 tablespoons chopped herbs (parsley, thyme, dill)
- ❖ 1 tablespoon olive oil
- ❖ Lemon wedges for serving

Instructions:

Mix breadcrumbs, herbs, and olive oil. Press onto halibut, bake until fish is cooked. Serve with lemon wedges.

Nutritional Info:

Calories: 250, Protein: 30g, Carbs: 5g, Fat: 10g

Cajun Grilled Tilapia

Servings: 2 | Prep Time: 5 mins | Cooking Time: 10 mins

Ingredients:

- ❖ 2 tilapia filets
- ❖ Cajun seasoning
- ❖ 1 tablespoon olive oil
- ❖ Lime wedges for serving

Instructions:

Rub tilapia with Cajun seasoning and olive oil. Grill until the fish flakes. Serve with lime wedges.

Nutritional Info:

Calories: 180, Protein: 25g, Carbs: 1g, Fat: 8g

Sesame Ginger Glazed Salmon

Servings: 2 | Prep Time: 10 mins | Cooking Time: 15 mins

Ingredients:

- ❖ 2 salmon filets
- ❖ 2 tablespoons soy sauce
- ❖ 1 tablespoon sesame oil
- ❖ 1 tablespoon honey

❖ 1 teaspoon grated ginger

Instructions:

Mix soy sauce, sesame oil, honey, and ginger. Marinate salmon, bake until done.

Nutritional Info:

Calories: 280, Protein: 30g, Carbs: 8g, Fat: 14g

Lemon Pepper Shrimp Skewers

Servings: 2 | Prep Time: 10 mins | Cooking Time: 5 mins

Ingredients:

❖ 1/2-pound large shrimp, peeled and deveined

❖ Zest and juice of 1 lemon

❖ 1 tablespoon olive oil

❖ 1 teaspoon black pepper

❖ Skewers for grilling

Instructions:

Marinate shrimp in lemon zest, juice, olive oil, and pepper. Skewer and grill until cooked.

Nutritional Info:

Calories: 200, Protein: 25g, Carbs: 2g, Fat: 10g

Garlic Lemon Butter Shrimp Pasta

Servings: 2 | Prep Time: 10 mins | Cooking Time: 15 mins

Ingredients:

- 1/2-pound shrimp, peeled and deveined

- 8 oz whole wheat pasta

- 2 tablespoons butter

- 2 cloves garlic, minced

- Juice of 1 lemon

- Fresh parsley for garnish

Instructions:

Cook pasta, reserve some pasta water. Sauté shrimp in butter and garlic, add lemon juice. Toss with pasta and a bit of pasta water. Garnish with parsley.

Nutritional Info:

Calories: 350, Protein: 25g, Carbs: 40g, Fat: 10g

Baked Cod with Tomato Basil Salsa

Servings: 2 | Prep Time: 10 mins | Cooking Time: 15 mins

Ingredients:

- 2 cod filets

- 1 cup cherry tomatoes, halved

- 2 tablespoons chopped basil

- 1 tablespoon olive oil

- Salt and pepper

Instructions:

Mix tomatoes, basil, olive oil, salt, and pepper. Top cod with the mixture, bake until fish flakes.

Nutritional Info:

Calories: 220, Protein: 30g, Carbs: 4g, Fat: 8g

Servings: 2 | Prep Time: 10 mins | Cooking Time: 15 mins

Coconut Lime Mahi Mahi

Servings: 2 | Prep Time: 10 mins | Cooking Time: 10 mins

Ingredients:

❖ 2 mahi mahi filets

❖ 1/4 cup coconut milk

❖ Zest and juice of 1 lime

❖ 1 tablespoon coconut oil

❖ Fresh cilantro for garnish

Instructions:

Mix coconut milk, lime zest, and juice. Marinate fish, pan-sear in coconut oil until cooked. Garnish with cilantro.

Nutritional Info:

Calories: 250, Protein: 30g, Carbs: 2g, Fat: 12g

Tuna Poke Bowl

Servings: 2 | Prep Time: 15 mins | Cooking Time: 0 mins

Ingredients:

❖ 1 cup cooked quinoa

❖ 1/2-pound sushi-grade tuna, cubed

❖ 1/4 cup soy sauce

❖ 1 tablespoon sesame oil

❖ Sliced cucumber, avocado, sesame seeds

Instructions:

Mix tuna with soy sauce and sesame oil. Serve over quinoa with cucumber, avocado, and sesame seeds.

Nutritional Info:

Calories: 320, Protein: 25g, Carbs: 20g, Fat: 15g

Lemon Garlic Shrimp Scampi

Servings: 2 | Prep Time: 10 mins | Cooking Time: 15 mins

Ingredients:

- ❖ 1/2-pound shrimp, peeled and deveined
- ❖ 8 oz whole wheat spaghetti
- ❖ 2 tablespoons olive oil
- ❖ 3 cloves garlic, minced
- ❖ Juice and zest of 1 lemon
- ❖ Red pepper flakes (optional)

Instructions:

Cook pasta, reserve some pasta water. Sauté shrimp and garlic in olive oil, add lemon juice, zest, and red pepper flakes. Toss with pasta and a bit of pasta water.

Nutritional Info:

Calories: 350, Protein: 25g, Carbs: 40g, Fat: 10g

Grilled Swordfish Steaks

Servings: 2 | Prep Time: 10 mins | Cooking Time: 10 mins

Ingredients:

- ❖ 2 swordfish steaks
- ❖ 2 tablespoons balsamic vinegar
- ❖ 1 tablespoon olive oil
- ❖ 1 teaspoon dried oregano
- ❖ Salt and pepper

Instructions:

Mix vinegar, olive oil, oregano, salt, and pepper. Marinate swordfish, grill until cooked.

Nutritional Info:

Calories: 300, Protein: 30g, Carbs: 2g, Fat: 15g

Baked Garlic Herb Salmon

Servings: 2 | Prep Time: 10 mins | Cooking Time: 15 mins

Ingredients:

- ❖ 2 salmon filets
- ❖ 2 tablespoons olive oil
- ❖ 2 cloves garlic, minced

* 1 tablespoon chopped herbs (rosemary, thyme)
* Lemon wedges for serving

Instructions:

Mix olive oil, garlic, and herbs. Rub onto salmon, bake until fish flakes. Serve with lemon wedges.

Nutritional Info:

Calories: 280, Protein: 30g, Carbs: 2g, Fat: 15g

Seared Scallops with Mango Salsa

Servings: 2 | Prep Time: 15 mins | Cooking Time: 5 mins

Ingredients:

* 1/2-pound scallops
* 1 mango, diced
* 1/4 cup red onion, finely chopped
* 1 jalapeño, seeded and diced
* Lime juice
* Fresh cilantro for garnish

Instructions:

Sear scallops until golden. Mix mango, onion, jalapeño, and lime juice for salsa. Serve scallops with salsa, garnish with cilantro.

Nutritional Info:

Calories: 250, Protein: 25g, Carbs: 20g, Fat: 8g

Honey Glazed Salmon

Servings: 2 | Prep Time: 10 mins | Cooking Time: 15 mins

Ingredients:

- ❖ 2 salmon filets
- ❖ 2 tablespoons honey
- ❖ 1 tablespoon soy sauce
- ❖ 1 tablespoon olive oil
- ❖ Sesame seeds for garnish

Instructions:

Mix honey, soy sauce, and olive oil. Brush onto salmon, bake until fish is cooked. Garnish with sesame seeds.

Nutritional Info:

Calories: 300, Protein: 30g, Carbs: 12g, Fat: 15g

Cajun Shrimp and Quinoa

Servings: 2 | Prep Time: 10 mins | Cooking Time: 10 mins

Ingredients:

- ❖ 1/2-pound shrimp, peeled and deveined
- ❖ 1 cup cooked quinoa
- ❖ Cajun seasoning
- ❖ 1 tablespoon olive oil
- ❖ Chopped green onions for garnish

Instructions:

Toss shrimp in Cajun seasoning. Sauté in olive oil until cooked. Serve over quinoa, garnish with green onions.

Nutritional Info:

Calories: 280, Protein: 25g, Carbs: 20g, Fat: 10g

Beans, Grains, and Pasta Recipes

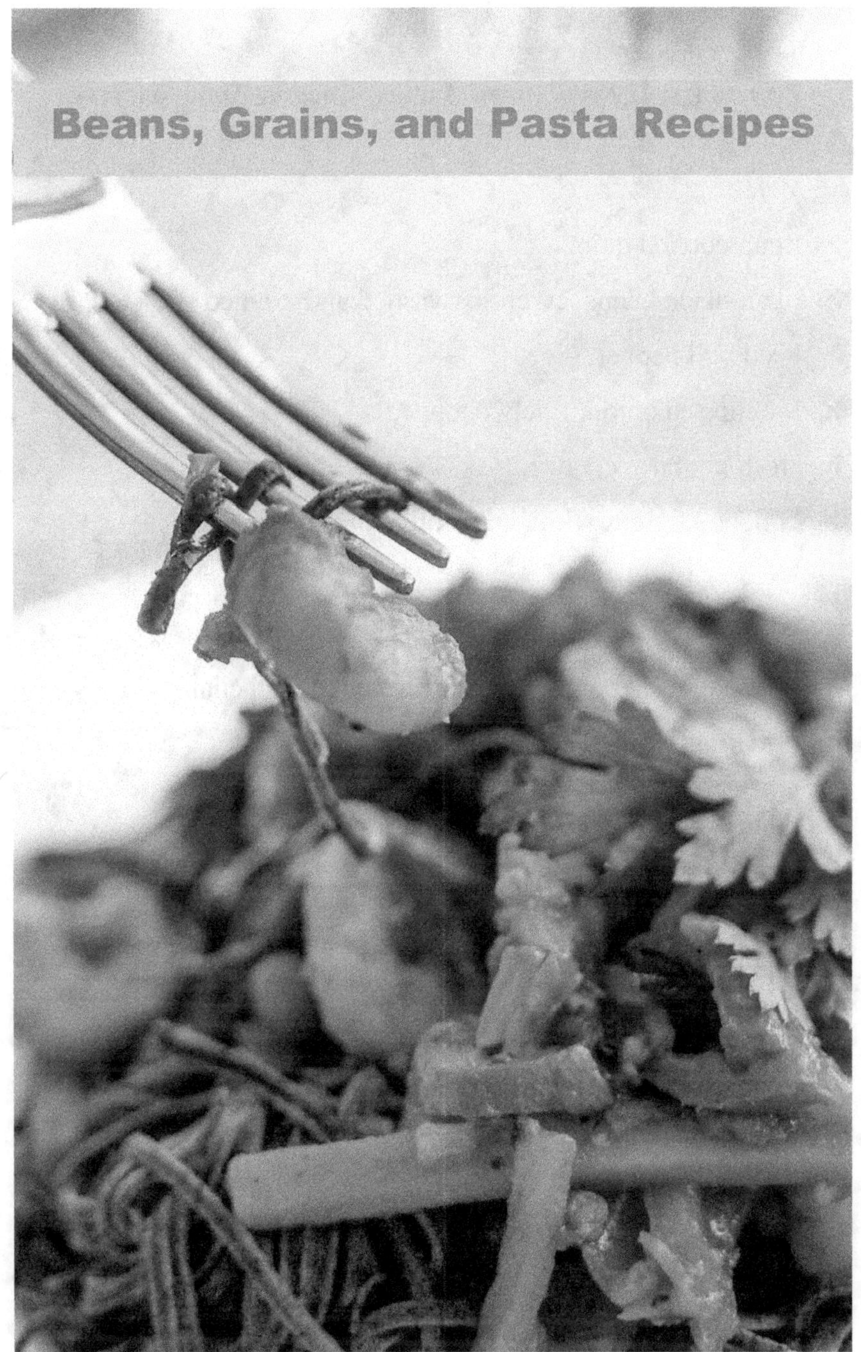

Black Bean Quinoa Salad

Servings: 2 | Prep Time: 15 mins | Cooking Time: 0 mins

Ingredients:

- ❖ 1 cup cooked quinoa
- ❖ 1 can black beans, carefully washed and drained
- ❖ 1 red bell pepper, diced
- ❖ 1/4 cup red onion, finely chopped
- ❖ Fresh cilantro, chopped
- ❖ Lime vinaigrette: lime juice, olive oil, salt, pepper

Instructions:

Mix quinoa, black beans, bell pepper, onion, and cilantro. Toss with lime vinaigrette.

Nutritional Info:

Calories: 280, Protein: 10g, Carbs: 45g, Fat: 8g

Lentil Curry

Servings: 2 | Prep Time: 10 mins | Cooking Time: 30 mins

Ingredients:

- ❖ 1 cup dried lentils
- ❖ 1 can coconut milk

- ❖ 1 onion, diced
- ❖ 2 cloves garlic, minced
- ❖ Curry powder, turmeric, cumin
- ❖ Spinach leaves

Instructions:

Cook lentils, sauté onion and garlic. Add cooked lentils, coconut milk, and spices. Simmer until flavors meld. Add spinach at the end.

Nutritional Info:

Calories: 320, Protein: 18g, Carbs: 40g, Fat: 10g

Chickpea Salad

Servings: 2 | Prep Time: 10 mins | Cooking Time: 0 mins

Ingredients:

- ❖ 1 can chickpeas, rinsed and drained
- ❖ 1 cucumber, diced
- ❖ 1 tomato, diced
- ❖ Red onion, thinly sliced
- ❖ Lemon vinaigrette: lemon juice, olive oil, salt, pepper, oregano

Instructions:

Combine chickpeas, cucumber, tomato, and onion. Toss with lemon vinaigrette.

Nutritional Info:

Calories: 250, Protein: 10g, Carbs: 35g, Fat: 10g

Spaghetti Aglio e Olio with Broccoli

Servings: 2 | Prep Time: 15 mins | Cooking Time: 15 mins

Ingredients:

- ❖ 8 oz whole wheat spaghetti
- ❖ 2 cups broccoli florets
- ❖ 4 cloves garlic, thinly sliced
- ❖ Red pepper flakes, olive oil
- ❖ Parmesan cheese for topping

Instructions:

Cook spaghetti, blanch broccoli. Sauté garlic and red pepper flakes in olive oil. Toss spaghetti and broccoli with garlic oil. Serve with Parmesan.

Nutritional Info:

Calories: 320, Protein: 12g, Carbs: 50g, Fat: 10g

Mediterranean Quinoa Bowl

Servings: 2 | Prep Time: 10 mins | Cooking Time: 0 mins

Ingredients:

- ❖ 1 cup cooked quinoa
- ❖ 1/2 cup cherry tomatoes, halved
- ❖ 1/2 cucumber, diced
- ❖ Kalamata olives, chopped
- ❖ Feta cheese crumbles
- ❖ Greek vinaigrette: red wine vinegar, olive oil, oregano

Instructions:

Combine quinoa, tomatoes, cucumber, olives, and feta. Drizzle with Greek vinaigrette.

Nutritional Info:

Calories: 300, Protein: 10g, Carbs: 35g, Fat: 15g

Red Lentil Soup

Servings: 2 | Prep Time: 10 mins | Cooking Time: 30 mins

Ingredients:

- ❖ 1 cup red lentils
- ❖ 1 onion, chopped

- ❖ 2 carrots, diced
- ❖ 2 cloves garlic, minced
- ❖ Vegetable broth
- ❖ Cumin, paprika, turmeric
- ❖ Fresh cilantro for garnish

Instructions:

Sauté onion, garlic, and carrots. Add lentils, spices, and broth. Simmer until the lentils are soft. Garnish with cilantro.

Nutritional Info:

Calories: 280, Protein: 15g, Carbs: 40g, Fat: 5g

Pasta Primavera

Servings: 2 | Prep Time: 15 mins | Cooking Time: 15 mins

Ingredients:

- ❖ 8 oz whole wheat pasta
- ❖ Assorted vegetables
- ❖ Garlic, olive oil, Italian herbs
- ❖ Parmesan cheese for topping

Instructions:

Cook pasta, sauté veggies and garlic in olive oil with herbs. Toss with pasta, serve with Parmesan.

Nutritional Info:

Calories: 350, Protein: 12g, Carbs: 60g, Fat: 10g

Mexican Black Bean Quinoa

Servings: 2 | Prep Time: 10 mins | Cooking Time: 0 mins

Ingredients:

- ❖ 1 cup cooked quinoa
- ❖ 1 can black beans, carefully washed and drained
- ❖ 1 bell pepper, diced
- ❖ Red onion, diced
- ❖ Salsa, lime juice, cilantro

Instructions:

Mix quinoa, black beans, bell pepper, and onion. Add salsa, lime juice, and cilantro for flavor.

Nutritional Info:

Calories: 290, Protein: 12g, Carbs: 45g, Fat: 5g

Pesto Pasta with Cherry Tomatoes

Servings: 2 | Prep Time: 10 mins | Cooking Time: 15 mins

Ingredients:

- ❖ 8 oz whole wheat spaghetti
- ❖ Pesto sauce (store-bought or homemade)
- ❖ Cherry tomatoes, halved
- ❖ Fresh basil leaves
- ❖ Pine nuts for topping

Instructions:

Cook pasta, toss with pesto sauce, cherry tomatoes, and basil. Top with pine nuts.

Nutritional Info:

Calories: 380, Protein: 10g, Carbs: 55g, Fat: 15g

Three Bean Salad

Servings: 2 | Prep Time: 10 mins | Cooking Time: 0 mins

Ingredients:

- ❖ 1 can kidney beans, drained
- ❖ 1 can garbanzo beans, drained
- ❖ 1 can green beans, drained

- ❖ Red onion, thinly sliced
- ❖ Italian dressing: red wine vinegar, olive oil, herbs

Instructions:

Combine beans and onion. Toss with Italian dressing.

Nutritional Info:

Calories: 260, Protein: 10g, Carbs: 35g, Fat: 10g

Butternut Squash and Lentil Curry

Servings: 2 | Prep Time: 15 mins | Cooking Time: 25 mins

Ingredients:

- ❖ 1 cup red lentils
- ❖ 2 cups butternut squash, diced
- ❖ 1 onion, chopped
- ❖ 2 cloves garlic, minced
- ❖ Curry paste, coconut milk
- ❖ Fresh cilantro for garnish

Instructions:

Sauté onion and garlic, add lentils, squash, curry paste, and coconut milk. Simmer until squash is tender. Garnish with cilantro.

Nutritional Info:

Calories: 290, Protein: 15g, Carbs: 40g, Fat: 8g

Pasta with Roasted Vegetables

Servings: 2 | Prep Time: 15 mins | Cooking Time: 25 mins

Ingredients:

- ❖ 8 oz whole wheat pasta
- ❖ Assorted vegetables (bell peppers, eggplant, onion)
- ❖ Olive oil, balsamic vinegar, Italian seasoning
- ❖ Parmesan cheese for topping

Instructions:

Roast vegetables tossed in olive oil, vinegar, and seasoning. Cook pasta, toss with roasted veggies. Serve with Parmesan.

Nutritional Info:

Calories: 360, Protein: 12g, Carbs: 60g, Fat: 10g

Quinoa Stuffed Bell Peppers

Servings: 2 | Prep Time: 15 mins | Cooking Time: 25 mins

Ingredients:

- ❖ 1 cup cooked quinoa

- ❖ 2 bell peppers, halved and seeded
- ❖ 1 can black beans, carefully washed and drained
- ❖ Corn, diced tomatoes, chili powder, cumin
- ❖ Shredded cheese for topping

Instructions:

Mix quinoa, black beans, corn, tomatoes, and spices. Stuff mixture into bell pepper halves. Top with cheese. Make sure to bake until peppers are tender.

Nutritional Info:

Calories: 280, Protein: 15g, Carbs: 40g, Fat: 8g

Spinach and Mushroom Risotto

Servings: 2 | Prep Time: 10 mins | Cooking Time: 30 mins

Ingredients:

- ❖ 1 cup Arborio rice
- ❖ 4 cups vegetable broth
- ❖ 1 onion, diced
- ❖ 2 cups mushrooms, sliced
- ❖ Fresh spinach, grated Parmesan

Instructions:

Sauté onion and mushrooms. Add rice, gradually stir in broth until absorbed. Stir in spinach, serve with Parmesan.

Nutritional Info:

Calories: 320, Protein: 8g, Carbs: 60g, Fat: 5g

Mediterranean Chickpea Pasta

Servings: 2 | Prep Time: 15 mins | Cooking Time: 15 mins

Ingredients:

- ❖ 8 oz whole wheat pasta
- ❖ 1 can chickpeas, carefully washed and drained
- ❖ Sun-dried tomatoes, olives, artichoke hearts
- ❖ Olive oil, lemon juice, garlic powder
- ❖ Fresh parsley for garnish

Instructions:

Cook pasta, mix with chickpeas, tomatoes, olives, artichokes. Dress with olive oil, lemon juice, and garlic powder. Garnish with parsley.

Nutritional Info:

Calories: 380, Protein: 15g, Carbs: 60g, Fat: 10g

Lentil and Vegetable Soup

Servings: 2 | Prep Time: 10 mins | Cooking Time: 30 mins

Ingredients:

- ❖ 1 cup green lentils
- ❖ 4 cups vegetable broth
- ❖ Carrots, celery, onion, diced
- ❖ 1 can diced tomatoes
- ❖ Italian herbs, bay leaves
- ❖ Fresh parsley for garnish

Instructions:

Sauté veggies, add lentils, broth, tomatoes, and herbs. Simmer until lentils are tender. Garnish with parsley.

Nutritional Info:

Calories: 250, Protein: 15g, Carbs: 40g, Fat: 5g

Spicy Black Bean Tacos

Servings: 2 | Prep Time: 10 mins | Cooking Time: 5 mins

Ingredients:

- ❖ 1 can black beans, mashed
- ❖ Taco shells or tortillas

- ❖ Sliced avocado, shredded lettuce, salsa
- ❖ Taco seasoning, lime juice, cilantro

Instructions:

Warm taco shells. Fill with mashed black beans, avocado, lettuce, salsa. Sprinkle it with taco seasoning, lime juice, and cilantro.

Nutritional Info:

Calories: 280, Protein: 10g, Carbs: 40g, Fat: 10g

Caprese Quinoa Salad

Servings: 2 | Prep Time: 10 mins | Cooking Time: 0 mins

Ingredients:

- ❖ 1 cup cooked quinoa
- ❖ Cherry tomatoes, mozzarella balls, fresh basil
- ❖ Balsamic glaze, olive oil, salt, pepper

Instructions:

Combine quinoa, tomatoes, mozzarella, and basil. Drizzle with balsamic glaze and olive oil. Season with salt and pepper.

Nutritional Info:

Calories: 300, Protein: 10g, Carbs: 30g, Fat: 15g

Pasta with White Bean and Tomato Sauce

Servings: 2 | Prep Time: 10 mins | Cooking Time: 15 mins

Ingredients:

- ❖ 8 oz whole wheat pasta
- ❖ 1 can white beans, carefully washed and drained
- ❖ Garlic, cherry tomatoes, spinach
- ❖ Olive oil, Italian herbs, red pepper flakes

Instructions:

Cook pasta, sauté garlic, add tomatoes, beans, and spinach. Toss with pasta, olive oil, herbs, and red pepper flakes.

Nutritional Info:

Calories: 340, Protein: 15g, Carbs: 60g, Fat: 5g

Butternut Squash and Chickpea Stew

Servings: 2 | Prep Time: 15 mins | Cooking Time: 25 mins

Ingredients:

- ❖ 2 cups butternut squash, cubed
- ❖ 1 can chickpeas, carefully washed and drained

- ❖ 1 onion, chopped
- ❖ 2 cloves garlic, minced
- ❖ Vegetable broth, cumin, paprika

Instructions:

Sauté onion and garlic, add squash, chickpeas, broth, and spices. Simmer until squash is tender.

Nutritional Info:

Calories: 280, Protein: 10g, Carbs: 50g, Fat: 5g

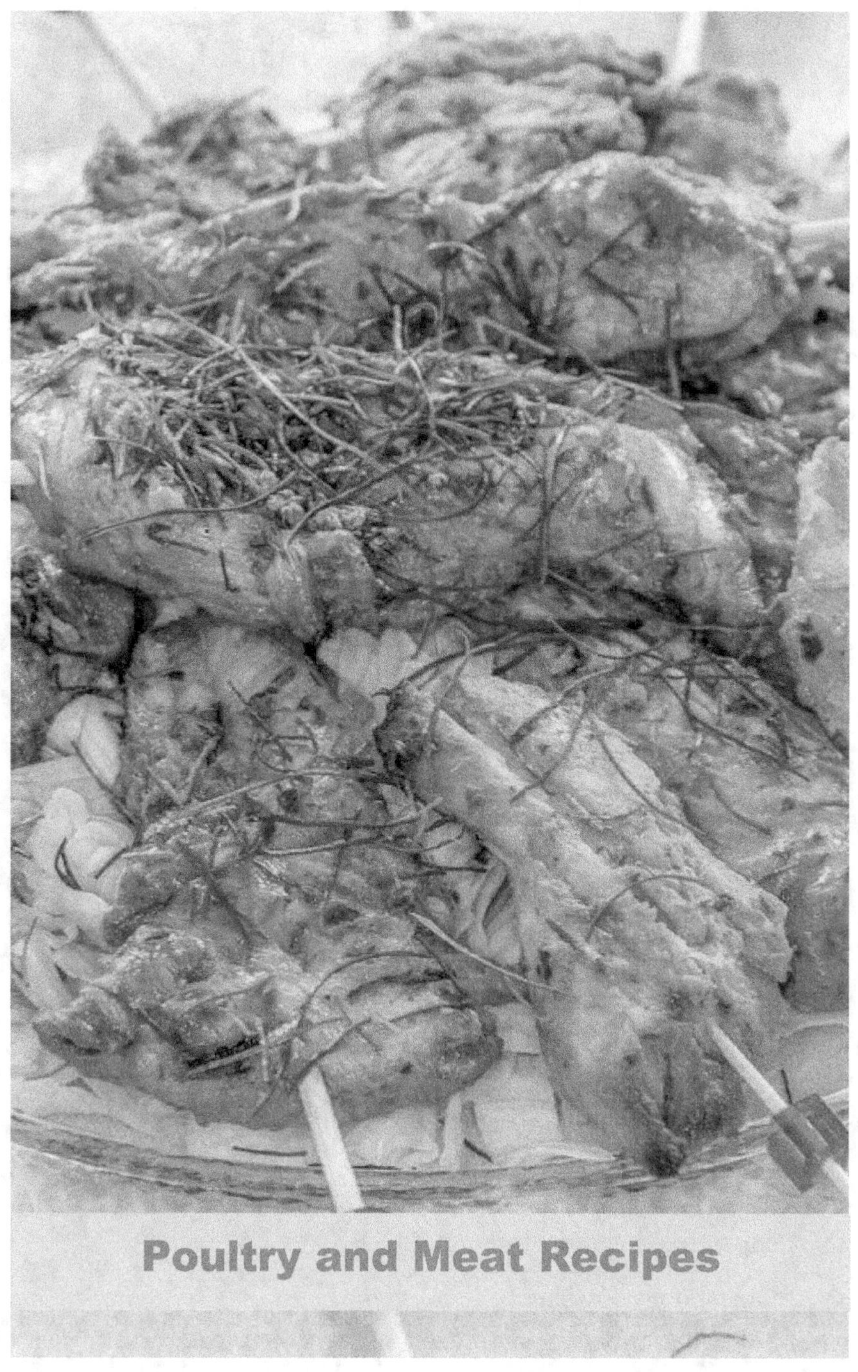
Poultry and Meat Recipes

Lemon Herb Chicken

Servings: 2 | Prep Time: 10 mins | Cooking Time: 20 mins

Ingredients:

- ❖ 2 chicken breasts
- ❖ 2 tablespoons olive oil
- ❖ 2 cloves garlic, minced
- ❖ Juice and zest of 1 lemon
- ❖ Fresh thyme, salt, pepper

Instructions:

Marinate chicken in olive oil, garlic, lemon zest, and thyme. Grill or bake until cooked. Season with salt, pepper, and lemon juice.

Nutritional Info:

Calories: 250, Protein: 30g, Carbs: 2g, Fat: 12g

Beef Stir-Fry

Servings: 2 | Prep Time: 15 mins | Cooking Time: 10 mins

Ingredients:

- ❖ 1/2-pound beef strips
- ❖ 2 cups mixed vegetables
- ❖ 2 tablespoons soy sauce

❖ 1 tablespoon sesame oil

❖ 1 clove garlic, minced

❖ Brown rice for serving

Instructions:

Stir-fry beef and veggies in sesame oil and garlic. Add soy sauce, cook until beef is done. Serve over brown rice.

Nutritional Info:

Calories: 300, Protein: 25g, Carbs: 15g, Fat: 12g

Turkey Meatballs in Marinara Sauce

Servings: 2 | Prep Time: 15 mins | Cooking Time: 20 mins

Ingredients:

❖ 1/2-pound ground turkey

❖ Bread crumbs, egg, grated onion, garlic powder

❖ Marinara sauce (store-bought or homemade)

❖ Fresh basil for garnish

Instructions:

Mix turkey, breadcrumbs, egg, onion, and garlic. Form into meatballs, bake. Serve with marinara sauce, garnish with basil.

Nutritional Info:

Calories: 220, Protein: 20g, Carbs: 10g, Fat: 10g

Balsamic Glazed Pork Chops

Servings: 2 | Prep Time: 10 mins | Cooking Time: 15 mins

Ingredients:

- ❖ 2 pork chops
- ❖ 2 tablespoons balsamic vinegar
- ❖ 1 tablespoon honey
- ❖ Dijon mustard, minced garlic
- ❖ Fresh rosemary, salt, pepper

Instructions:

Mix balsamic vinegar, honey, mustard, garlic, and rosemary. Marinate pork chops, grill or bake until cooked. Season with salt and pepper.

Nutritional Info:

Calories: 280, Protein: 25g, Carbs: 10g, Fat: 15g

Chicken and Vegetable Skewers

Servings: 2 | Prep Time: 15 mins | Cooking Time: 10 mins

Ingredients:

- 2 chicken breasts, cubed

- Assorted vegetables (bell peppers, onions, zucchini)

- Olive oil, lemon juice, garlic powder

- Skewers for grilling

Instructions:

Thread chicken and veggies on skewers. Mix olive oil, lemon juice, and garlic powder. Grill until chicken is cooked.

Nutritional Info:

Calories: 240, Protein: 30g, Carbs: 10g, Fat: 10g

Honey Mustard Glazed Salmon

Servings: 2 | Prep Time: 10 mins | Cooking Time: 15 mins

Ingredients:

- ❖ 2 salmon filets

- ❖ 2 tablespoons honey

- ❖ 1 tablespoon Dijon mustard

- ❖ 1 tablespoon olive oil

❖ Fresh dill for garnish

Instructions:

Mix honey, mustard, and olive oil. Brush onto salmon, bake until fish flakes. Garnish with fresh dill.

Nutritional Info:

Calories: 280, Protein: 30g, Carbs: 10g, Fat: 15g

Lemon Garlic Turkey Cutlets

Servings: 2 | Prep Time: 10 mins | Cooking Time: 10 mins

Ingredients:

❖ 2 turkey cutlets

❖ 2 tablespoons olive oil

❖ 2 cloves garlic, minced

❖ Juice and zest of 1 lemon

❖ Fresh parsley, salt, pepper

Instructions:

Marinate turkey in olive oil, garlic, lemon zest, and juice. Pan-sear until cooked. Season with parsley, salt, and pepper.

Nutritional Info:

Calories: 220, Protein: 25g, Carbs: 2g, Fat: 12g

Teriyaki Chicken Stir-Fry

Servings: 2 | Prep Time: 15 mins | Cooking Time: 10 mins

Ingredients:

- ❖ 2 chicken thighs, sliced
- ❖ 2 cups mixed vegetables (snap peas, bell peppers, carrots)
- ❖ 2 tablespoons teriyaki sauce
- ❖ 1 tablespoon sesame oil
- ❖ 1 clove garlic, minced
- ❖ Jasmine rice for serving

Instructions:

Stir-fry chicken and veggies in sesame oil and garlic. Add teriyaki sauce, cook until chicken is done. Serve over jasmine rice.

Nutritional Info:

Calories: 320, Protein: 20g, Carbs: 30g, Fat: 12g

Beef and Broccoli

Servings: 2 | Prep Time: 15 mins | Cooking Time: 10 mins

Ingredients:

- ❖ 1/2-pound beef strips
- ❖ 2 cups broccoli florets
- ❖ 2 tablespoons soy sauce
- ❖ 1 tablespoon brown sugar
- ❖ 1 clove garlic, minced
- ❖ Brown rice for serving

Instructions:

Sauté beef and broccoli, add soy sauce, brown sugar, and garlic. Cook until beef is done. Serve over brown rice.

Nutritional Info:

Calories: 300, Protein: 25g, Carbs: 20g, Fat: 12g

Lemon Rosemary Grilled Chicken

Servings: 2 | Prep Time: 10 mins | Cooking Time: 15 mins

Ingredients:

- ❖ 2 chicken thighs
- ❖ 2 tablespoons olive oil

- ❖ 2 cloves garlic, minced
- ❖ Juice and zest of 1 lemon
- ❖ Fresh rosemary, salt, pepper

Instructions:

Marinate chicken in olive oil, garlic, lemon zest, juice, and rosemary. Grill until cooked. Season with salt and pepper.

Nutritional Info:

Calories: 250, Protein: 25g, Carbs: 2g, Fat: 15g

Turkey Sausage and Peppers

Servings: 2 | Prep Time: 10 mins | Cooking Time: 20 mins

Ingredients:

- ❖ 4 turkey sausage links, sliced
- ❖ 2 bell peppers, sliced
- ❖ 1 onion, sliced
- ❖ 1 can diced tomatoes
- ❖ Italian seasoning, red pepper flakes

Instructions:

Sauté sausage, peppers, and onion. Add diced tomatoes and seasonings. Simmer until flavors meld.

Nutritional Info:

Calories: 280, Protein: 20g, Carbs: 15g, Fat: 15g

Herb-Crusted Pork Tenderloin

Servings: 2 | Prep Time: 10 mins | Cooking Time: 25 mins

Ingredients:

- ❖ 1 pork tenderloin
- ❖ 2 tablespoons Dijon mustard
- ❖ Bread crumbs, chopped herbs (rosemary, thyme)
- ❖ Garlic powder, salt, pepper

Instructions:

Coat pork with Dijon mustard, herb mixture, garlic powder, salt, and pepper. Roast until cooked.

Nutritional Info:

Calories: 260, Protein: 30g, Carbs: 5g, Fat: 12g

Chicken Fajitas

Servings: 2 | Prep Time: 15 mins | Cooking Time: 10 mins

Ingredients:

- ❖ 2 chicken breasts, sliced

- ❖ Bell peppers, onion, sliced
- ❖ Fajita seasoning
- ❖ Tortillas, sliced avocado, salsa

Instructions:

Sauté chicken, peppers, and onions with fajita seasoning. You can serve in tortillas with avocado and salsa.

Nutritional Info:

Calories: 300, Protein: 25g, Carbs: 25g, Fat: 12g

Italian Herb Grilled Steak

Servings: 2 | Prep Time: 10 mins | Cooking Time: 15 mins

Ingredients:

- ❖ 2 beef steaks
- ❖ 2 tablespoons olive oil
- ❖ Italian herbs, minced garlic
- ❖ Balsamic vinegar
- ❖ Salt, pepper

Instructions:

Marinate steaks in olive oil, herbs, garlic, and balsamic vinegar. Grill until desired doneness. Season with salt and pepper.

Nutritional Info:

Calories: 300, Protein: 25g, Carbs: 2g, Fat: 20g

Honey Lime Chicken Skewers

Servings: 2 | Prep Time: 15 mins | Cooking Time: 10 mins

Ingredients:

- ❖ 2 chicken breasts, cubed
- ❖ 2 tablespoons honey
- ❖ Juice and zest of 1 lime
- ❖ Soy sauce, garlic powder
- ❖ Wooden skewers

Instructions:

Mix honey, lime juice, zest, soy sauce, and garlic powder. Thread chicken onto skewers. Grill until cooked.

Nutritional Info:

Calories: 240, Protein: 30g, Carbs: 10g, Fat: 8g

BBQ Glazed Pork Chops

Servings: 2 | Prep Time: 10 mins | Cooking Time: 20 mins

Ingredients:

- ❖ 2 pork chops
- ❖ BBQ sauce
- ❖ 1 tablespoon olive oil
- ❖ Paprika, garlic powder, salt, pepper

Instructions:

Rub pork chops with paprika, garlic powder, salt, and pepper. Grill or bake, baste with BBQ sauce.

Nutritional Info:

Calories: 280, Protein: 30g, Carbs: 15g, Fat: 12g

Lemon Garlic Herb Turkey Cutlets

Servings: 2 | Prep Time: 10 mins | Cooking Time: 10 mins

Ingredients:

- ❖ 2 turkey cutlets
- ❖ 2 tablespoons olive oil
- ❖ 2 cloves garlic, minced
- ❖ Juice and zest of 1 lemon

❖ Fresh thyme, salt, pepper

Instructions:

Marinate turkey in olive oil, garlic, lemon zest, juice, and thyme. Pan-sear until cooked. Season with salt and pepper.

Nutritional Info:

Calories: 230, Protein: 25g, Carbs: 2g, Fat: 14g

Moroccan Spiced Chicken

Servings: 2 | Prep Time: 10 mins | Cooking Time: 15 mins

Ingredients:

❖ 2 chicken thighs
❖ Moroccan spice blend (cumin, paprika, coriander)
❖ 2 tablespoons olive oil
❖ Lemon wedges for serving

Instructions:

Coat chicken with Moroccan spices and olive oil. Grill or bake until done. Serve with lemon wedges.

Nutritional Info:

Calories: 260, Protein: 25g, Carbs: 2g, Fat: 15g

Vegan and Vegetarian Recipes

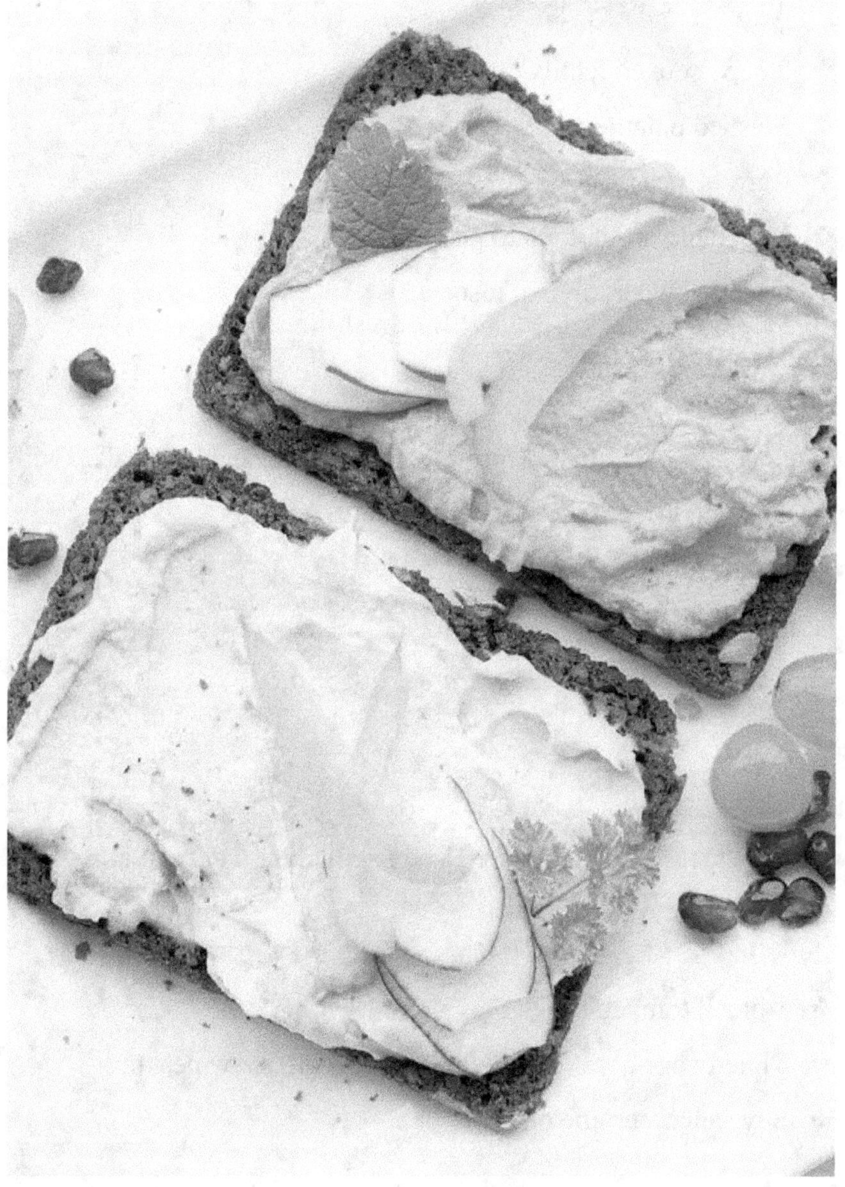

Lentil Shepherd's Pie

Servings: 2 | Prep Time: 20 mins | Cooking Time: 25 mins

Ingredients:

- ❖ 2 cups cooked lentils
- ❖ Mashed potatoes
- ❖ Carrots, peas, onions
- ❖ Vegetable broth, tomato paste
- ❖ Garlic powder, thyme, rosemary

Instructions:

Sauté veggies, add lentils, broth, tomato paste, and herbs. Top with mashed potatoes. Make sure to bake until golden.

Nutritional Info:

Calories: 320, Protein: 15g, Carbs: 50g, Fat: 5g

Tofu Stir-Fry

Servings: 2 | Prep Time: 15 mins | Cooking Time: 10 mins

Ingredients:

- ❖ 1 block tofu, cubed
- ❖ Mixed vegetables (bell peppers, broccoli, snow peas)
- ❖ Soy sauce, sesame oil

❖ Ginger, garlic, red pepper flakes

Instructions:

Stir-fry tofu and veggies in sesame oil, ginger, garlic, and soy sauce. Sprinkle it with red pepper flakes.

Nutritional Info:

Calories: 280, Protein: 20g, Carbs: 15g, Fat: 15g

Vegan Chili

Servings: 2 | Prep Time: 10 mins | Cooking Time: 25 mins

Ingredients:

❖ 1 can kidney beans
❖ 1 can black beans
❖ 1 can diced tomatoes
❖ Bell peppers, onions, corn
❖ Chili powder, cumin, paprika

Instructions:

Sauté veggies, add beans, tomatoes, and spices. Simmer until flavors meld.

Nutritional Info:

Calories: 290, Protein: 15g, Carbs: 50g, Fat: 5g

Eggplant and Chickpea Tagine

Servings: 2 | Prep Time: 15 mins | Cooking Time: 25 mins

Ingredients:

- ❖ 1 eggplant, diced
- ❖ 1 can chickpeas, carefully washed and drained
- ❖ Tomatoes, onions, garlic
- ❖ Vegetable broth, cumin, cinnamon

Instructions:

Sauté veggies, add chickpeas, tomatoes, broth, and spices. Simmer until the eggplant is tender.

Nutritional Info:

Calories: 250, Protein: 10g, Carbs: 40g, Fat: 5g

Vegan Pasta Primavera

Servings: 2 | Prep Time: 15 mins | Cooking Time: 15 mins

Ingredients:

- ❖ 8 oz whole wheat pasta

- ❖ Assorted vegetables
- ❖ Garlic, olive oil, Italian herbs

Instructions:

Sauté veggies and garlic in olive oil with Italian herbs. Toss with cooked pasta.

Nutritional Info:

Calories: 320, Protein: 10g, Carbs: 60g, Fat: 5g

Quinoa and Vegetable Stuffed Peppers

Servings: 2 | Prep Time: 15 mins | Cooking Time: 25 mins

Ingredients:

- ❖ 1 cup cooked quinoa
- ❖ Bell peppers
- ❖ Mixed vegetables
- ❖ Tomato sauce, Italian seasoning

Instructions:

Mix quinoa, veggies, tomato sauce, and seasoning. Stuff into bell peppers, bake until peppers are tender.

Nutritional Info:

Calories: 280, Protein: 8g, Carbs: 50g, Fat: 5g

Vegan Lentil Sloppy Joes

Servings: 2 | Prep Time: 10 mins | Cooking Time: 15 mins

Ingredients:

- ❖ 1 cup cooked lentils
- ❖ Onion, bell pepper, garlic
- ❖ Tomato sauce, Dijon mustard, maple syrup
- ❖ Hamburger buns

Instructions:

Sauté veggies, add lentils, tomato sauce, mustard, and syrup. Serve on hamburger buns.

Nutritional Info:

Calories: 290, Protein: 15g, Carbs: 45g, Fat: 5g

Sweet Potato Black Bean Enchiladas

Servings: 2 | Prep Time: 10 mins | Cooking Time: 15 mins

Ingredients:

- ❖ 2 sweet potatoes, mashed
- ❖ 1 can black beans, carefully washed and drained
- ❖ Corn tortillas
- ❖ Enchilada sauce, cumin, chili powder

Instructions:

Mix sweet potatoes, beans, and spices. Roll into tortillas, top with enchilada sauce, bake until bubbly.

Nutritional Info:

Calories: 300, Protein: 10g, Carbs: 50g, Fat: 5g

Vegan Chickpea Curry

Servings: 2 | Prep Time: 15 mins | Cooking Time: 25 mins

Ingredients:

- ❖ 1 can chickpeas, carefully washed and drained
- ❖ Tomatoes, onions, garlic
- ❖ Coconut milk, curry powder, turmeric

Instructions:

Sauté veggies, add chickpeas, tomatoes, coconut milk, and spices. Simmer until flavors blend.

Nutritional Info:

Calories: 280, Protein: 12g, Carbs: 40g, Fat: 10g

Vegan Mushroom Stroganoff

Servings: 2 | Prep Time: 15 mins | Cooking Time: 20 mins

Ingredients:

- ❖ 8 oz mushrooms, sliced
- ❖ Onion, garlic
- ❖ Vegetable broth, soy sauce, flour
- ❖ Dairy-free sour cream
- ❖ Whole wheat pasta

Instructions:

Sauté mushrooms, onion, and garlic. Add broth, soy sauce, and flour to thicken. Stir in dairy-free sour cream, serve over pasta.

Nutritional Info:

Calories: 320, Protein: 10g, Carbs: 60g, Fat: 5g

Vegan Quinoa Buddha Bowl

Servings: 2 | Prep Time: 20 mins | Cooking Time: 25 mins

Ingredients:

- ❖ 1 cup cooked quinoa
- ❖ Assorted vegetables
- ❖ Avocado, tahini dressing

Instructions:

Arrange quinoa and veggies in a bowl. Nicely and gently top with sliced avocado and drizzle with tahini dressing.

Nutritional Info:

Calories: 350, Protein: 10g, Carbs: 45g, Fat: 15g

Vegan Chickpea Salad Sandwich

Servings: 2 | Prep Time: 10 mins | Cooking Time: 0 mins

Ingredients:

- ❖ 1 can chickpeas, mashed
- ❖ Celery, red onion, pickles
- ❖ Vegan mayo, Dijon mustard
- ❖ Whole grain bread

Instructions:

Mix chickpeas, veggies, mayo, and mustard. Spread on bread to make sandwiches.

Nutritional Info:

Calories: 280, Protein: 10g, Carbs: 45g, Fat: 8g

Vegan Spinach and Artichoke Pasta

Servings: 2 | Prep Time: 15 mins | Cooking Time: 15 mins

Ingredients:

- ❖ 8 oz whole wheat pasta
- ❖ Spinach, artichoke hearts
- ❖ Cashew cream sauce
- ❖ Nutritional yeast for topping

Instructions:

Cook pasta, sauté spinach and artichokes. Toss with cashew cream sauce, sprinkle with nutritional yeast.

Nutritional Info:

Calories: 340, Protein: 10g, Carbs: 60g, Fat: 8g

Vegan Black Bean Burgers

Servings: 2 | Prep Time: 15 mins | Cooking Time: 15 mins

Ingredients:

- ❖ 1 can black beans, mashed
- ❖ Bread crumbs, oats, flaxseed meal
- ❖ Onion, garlic, spices
- ❖ Whole grain burger buns

Instructions:

Mix mashed beans, bread crumbs, oats, flaxseed, onion, garlic, and spices. Form into patties, grill or bake.

Nutritional Info:

Calories: 290, Protein: 12g, Carbs: 50g, Fat: 5g

Vegan Cauliflower Curry

Servings: 2 | Prep Time: 15 mins | Cooking Time: 25 mins

Ingredients:

- ❖ 1 head cauliflower, chopped
- ❖ Tomatoes, onions, garlic
- ❖ Coconut milk, curry powder, turmeric

Instructions:

Sauté veggies, add cauliflower, tomatoes, coconut milk, and spices. Simmer until the cauliflower is tender.

Nutritional Info:

Calories: 260, Protein: 8g, Carbs: 40g, Fat: 10g

Vegan Lentil Meatballs

Servings: 2 | Prep Time: 15 mins | Cooking Time: 20 mins

Ingredients:

- ❖ 1 cup cooked lentils
- ❖ Bread crumbs, oats, flaxseed meal
- ❖ Onion, garlic, Italian seasoning
- ❖ Marinara sauce

Instructions:

Mix lentils, bread crumbs, oats, flaxseed, onion, garlic, and seasoning. Form into balls, bake. Serve with marinara.

Nutritional Info:

Calories: 280, Protein: 12g, Carbs: 40g, Fat: 8g

Vegan Ratatouille

Servings: 2 | Prep Time: 20 mins | Cooking Time: 30 mins

Ingredients:

- ❖ Eggplant, zucchini, tomatoes
- ❖ Bell peppers, onions, garlic
- ❖ Fresh herbs (thyme, rosemary)
- ❖ Olive oil, balsamic vinegar

Instructions:

Layer sliced veggies in a dish, drizzle with olive oil, herbs, and vinegar. Bake until tender.

Nutritional Info:

Calories: 240, Protein: 8g, Carbs: 40g, Fat: 8g

Vegan Sweet Potato and Black Bean Chili

Servings: 2 | Prep Time: 15 mins | Cooking Time: 25 mins

Ingredients:

- ❖ 1 sweet potato, diced
- ❖ 1 can black beans
- ❖ Bell peppers, onions, garlic

* Vegetable broth, chili powder, cumin

Instructions:

Sauté veggies, add sweet potato, beans, broth, and spices. Simmer until the sweet potato is tender.

Nutritional Info:

Calories: 280, Protein: 10g, Carbs: 50g, Fat: 5g

Vegan Mushroom and Spinach Quesadillas

Servings: 2 | Prep Time: 10 mins | Cooking Time: 10 mins

Ingredients:

* Whole wheat tortillas
* Mushrooms, spinach
* Vegan cheese, nutritional yeast
* Avocado for serving

Instructions:

Fill tortillas with mushrooms, spinach, vegan cheese, and nutritional yeast. Grill until crispy. Serve with avocado.

Nutritional Info:

Calories: 320, Protein: 10g, Carbs: 45g, Fat: 10g

Vegan Lentil and Spinach Curry

Servings: 2 | Prep Time: 15 mins | Cooking Time: 25 mins

Ingredients:

- ❖ 1 cup cooked lentils
- ❖ Spinach, tomatoes, onions
- ❖ Coconut milk, curry powder, turmeric

Instructions:

Sauté veggies, add lentils, tomatoes, coconut milk, and spices. Simmer until flavors meld.

Nutritional Info:

Calories: 270, Protein: 12g, Carbs: 40g, Fat: 8g

Vegan Cauliflower Tacos

Servings: 2 | Prep Time: 10 mins | Cooking Time: 25 mins

Ingredients:

- ❖ 1 head cauliflower, florets
- ❖ Taco seasoning

* ❖ Tortillas, sliced avocado, salsa
* ❖ Lime wedges for serving

Instructions:

Toss cauliflower with taco seasoning. Roast until tender. Make sure to serve in tortillas with avocado, salsa, and lime wedges.

Nutritional Info:

Calories: 290, Protein: 8g, Carbs: 45g, Fat: 10g

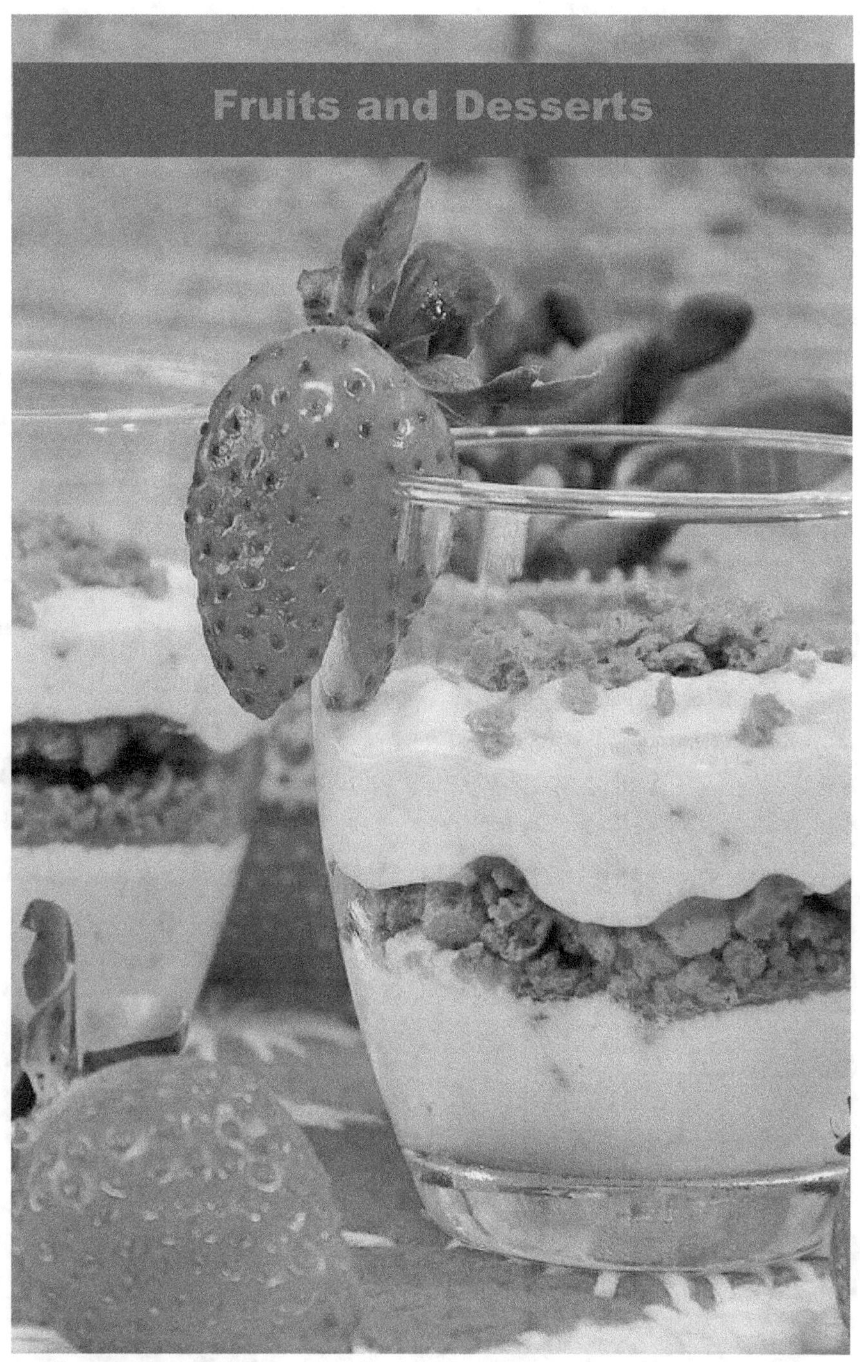
Fruits and Desserts

Mixed Berry Smoothie Bowl

Servings: 2 | Prep Time: 10 mins | Cooking Time: 0 mins

Ingredients:

- ❖ Mixed berries (strawberries, blueberries, raspberries)
- ❖ Banana, almond milk
- ❖ Toppings: granola, shredded coconut, chia seeds

Instructions:

Blend berries, banana, and almond milk until smooth. Gently transfer into a bowl, top with granola, coconut, and chia seeds.

Nutritional Info:

Calories: 250, Protein: 5g, Carbs: 50g, Fat: 5g

Apple Cinnamon Oatmeal

Servings: 2 | Prep Time: 5 mins | Cooking Time: 10 mins

Ingredients:

- ❖ Rolled oats
- ❖ Apples, cinnamon
- ❖ Almond milk, maple syrup
- ❖ Chopped nuts for topping

Instructions:

Cook oats with chopped apples, cinnamon, almond milk, and maple syrup. Top with chopped nuts.

Nutritional Info:

Calories: 280, Protein: 7g, Carbs: 50g, Fat: 8g

Banana Walnut Pancakes

Servings: 2 | Prep Time: 10 mins | Cooking Time: 15 mins

Ingredients:

- ❖ Whole wheat flour
- ❖ Mashed ripe bananas
- ❖ Chopped walnuts, almond milk
- ❖ Baking powder, vanilla extract

Instructions:

Mix flour, bananas, walnuts, almond milk, baking powder, and vanilla. Cook as pancakes.

Nutritional Info:

Calories: 320, Protein: 9g, Carbs: 50g, Fat: 10g

Peach and Blueberry Cobbler

Servings: 2 | Prep Time: 15 mins | Cooking Time: 25 mins

Ingredients:

- ❖ Fresh peaches, blueberries
- ❖ Whole wheat flour, oats
- ❖ Maple syrup, cinnamon
- ❖ Coconut oil, almond milk

Instructions:

Mix peaches, blueberries, flour, oats, syrup, cinnamon, and almond milk. Bake until bubbly.

Nutritional Info:

Calories: 280, Protein: 5g, Carbs: 50g, Fat: 8g

Mixed Fruit Salad

Servings: 2 | Prep Time: 10 mins | Cooking Time: 0 mins

Ingredients:

- ❖ Assorted fruits (strawberries, pineapple, grapes)
- ❖ Mint leaves
- ❖ Honey, lime juice

Instructions:

Combine fruits, mint leaves, honey, and lime juice in a bowl. Toss gently and serve.

Nutritional Info:

Calories: 150, Protein: 2g, Carbs: 35g, Fat: 1g

Watermelon Lime Popsicles

Servings: 4 | Prep Time: 10 mins | Cooking Time: 0 mins

Ingredients:

- ❖ Fresh watermelon chunks
- ❖ Lime juice, honey
- ❖ Popsicle molds

Instructions:

Blend watermelon, lime juice, and honey. Pour into popsicle molds, freeze until solid.

Nutritional Info:

Calories: 60, Protein: 1g, Carbs: 15g, Fat: 0g

Coconut Mango Rice Pudding

Servings: 2 | Prep Time: 5 mins | Cooking Time: 20 mins

Ingredients:

- ❖ Cooked rice
- ❖ Coconut milk, diced mango
- ❖ Maple syrup, shredded coconut

Instructions:

Mix rice, coconut milk, mango, and maple syrup. Simmer until creamy. Top with shredded coconut.

Nutritional Info:

Calories: 280, Protein: 4g, Carbs: 50g, Fat: 8g

Berry Chia Seed Pudding

Servings: 2 | Prep Time: 5 mins | Cooking Time: 0 mins

Ingredients:

- ❖ Chia seeds
- ❖ Almond milk
- ❖ Mixed berries (strawberries, raspberries)
- ❖ Maple syrup

Instructions:

Mix chia seeds, almond milk, berries, and maple syrup. Chill overnight until pudding-like consistency.

Nutritional Info:

Calories: 220, Protein: 5g, Carbs: 30g, Fat: 10g

Pineapple Coconut Sorbet

Servings: 2 | Prep Time: 10 mins | Cooking Time: 0 mins

Ingredients:

- ❖ Fresh pineapple chunks
- ❖ Coconut milk
- ❖ Lime zest, shredded coconut

Instructions:

Blend pineapple, coconut milk, and lime zest until smooth. Freeze until firm. Serve topped with shredded coconut.

Nutritional Info:

Calories: 180, Protein: 2g, Carbs: 30g, Fat: 8g

Avocado Chocolate Mousse

Servings: 2 | Prep Time: 5 mins | Cooking Time: 0 mins

Ingredients:

❖ Ripe avocados

❖ Cocoa powder

❖ Maple syrup, vanilla extract

Instructions:

Blend avocados, cocoa powder, maple syrup, and vanilla until smooth. Chill before serving.

Nutritional Info:

Calories: 250, Protein: 3g, Carbs: 20g, Fat: 18g

Banana Chocolate Chip Muffins

Servings: 2 | Prep Time: 10 mins | Cooking Time: 20 mins

Ingredients:

❖ Whole wheat flour

❖ Mashed ripe bananas

❖ Chocolate chips, almond milk

❖ Baking powder, cinnamon

Instructions:

Mix flour, bananas, chocolate chips, almond milk, baking powder, and cinnamon. Bake as muffins.

Nutritional Info:

Calories: 240, Protein: 5g, Carbs: 40g, Fat: 8g

Raspberry Coconut Popsicles

Servings: 4 | Prep Time: 10 mins | Cooking Time: 0 mins

Ingredients:

- ❖ Fresh raspberries
- ❖ Coconut water
- ❖ Agave syrup

Instructions:

Blend raspberries, coconut water, and agave syrup. Pour into popsicle molds, freeze until solid.

Nutritional Info:

Calories: 60, Protein: 1g, Carbs: 15g, Fat: 0g

Lemon Blueberry Scones

Servings: 2 | Prep Time: 10 mins | Cooking Time: 20 mins

Ingredients:

- ❖ Whole wheat flour
- ❖ Fresh blueberries
- ❖ Lemon zest, almond milk
- ❖ Maple syrup

Instructions:

Mix flour, blueberries, lemon zest, almond milk, and maple syrup. Bake as scones.

Nutritional Info:

Calories: 220, Protein: 5g, Carbs: 40g, Fat: 5g

Mango Coconut Rice Pudding

Servings: 2 | Prep Time: 5 mins | Cooking Time: 20 mins

Ingredients:

- ❖ Cooked rice
- ❖ Coconut milk
- ❖ Diced mango, shredded coconut
- ❖ Agave syrup

Instructions:

Mix rice, coconut milk, mango, shredded coconut, and agave syrup. Simmer until creamy.

Nutritional Info:

Calories: 270, Protein: 3g, Carbs: 50g, Fat: 8g

Strawberry Banana Parfait

Servings: 2 | Prep Time: 10 mins | Cooking Time: 0 mins

Ingredients:

- ❖ Fresh strawberries, sliced
- ❖ Ripe bananas, sliced
- ❖ Greek yogurt or coconut yogurt
- ❖ Granola

Instructions:

Layer strawberries, bananas, and yogurt in glasses. Top with granola.

Nutritional Info:

Calories: 220, Protein: 7g, Carbs: 40g, Fat: 5g

Apple Cinnamon Bread

Servings: 2 | Prep Time: 10 mins | Cooking Time: 30 mins

Ingredients:

- ❖ Whole wheat flour
- ❖ Chopped apples
- ❖ Cinnamon, nutmeg
- ❖ Maple syrup, almond milk

Instructions:

Mix flour, apples, cinnamon, nutmeg, maple syrup, and almond milk. Bake as bread.

Nutritional Info:

Calories: 250, Protein: 5g, Carbs: 40g, Fat: 5g

30-DAY

MEAL

PLAN

KEY

A-BREAKFAST

B-LUNCH

C-DINNER

DAY	A	B	C
1	Mixed Berry Smoothie Bowl	Greek Salad with Grilled Chicken	Baked Salmon with Asparagus
2	Apple Cinnamon Oatmeal	Lentil Soup with Whole Wheat Bread	Quinoa and Vegetable Stir-Fry
3	Banana Walnut Pancakes	Tofu Stir-Fry	Lentil Shepherd's Pie
4	Peach and Blueberry Cobbler	Chicken Fajitas	Eggplant and Chickpea Tagine
5	Mixed Fruit Salad	Vegan Chili	Italian Herb Grilled Steak

DAY	A	B	C
6	Watermelon Lime Popsicles	BBQ Glazed Pork Chops	Vegan Pasta Primavera
7	Coconut Mango Rice Pudding	Lemon Garlic Herb Turkey Cutlets	Sweet Potato Black Bean Enchiladas
8	Berry Chia Seed Pudding	Moroccan Spiced Chicken	Vegan Lentil Sloppy Joes
9	Avocado Chocolate Mousse	Mushroom and Spinach Quesadillas	Lentil and Spinach Curry
10	Banana Chocolate Chip Muffins	Vegan Chickpea Curry	Moroccan Spiced Salmon

DAY	A	B	C
11	Raspberry Coconut Popsicles	Chicken Caesar Salad	Vegan Cauliflower Curry
12	Lemon Blueberry Scones	Caprese Salad with Grilled Chicken	Vegan Ratatouille
13	Mango Coconut Rice Pudding	Black Bean and Corn Salad	Honey Lime Chicken Skewers
14	Strawberry Banana Parfait	Lentil and Vegetable Stir-Fry	Grilled Swordfish with Quinoa Salad
15	Apple Cinnamon Bread	Chickpea and Avocado Salad	Greek Lemon Chicken with Roasted Vegetables

DAY	A	B	C
16	Mixed Berry Smoothie Bowl	Italian Vegetable Soup with Whole Wheat Bread	Baked Cod with Lemon and Garlic
17	Lentil Soup with Whole Wheat Bread	Greek Salad with Grilled Chicken	Vegan Mushroom Stroganoff
18	Banana Walnut Pancakes	Tofu Stir-Fry	Lentil Shepherd's Pie
19	Peach and Blueberry Cobbler	Chicken Fajitas	Eggplant and Chickpea Tagine
20	Mixed Fruit Salad	Vegan Chili	Italian Herb Grilled Steak

DAY	A	B	C
21	Watermelon Lime Popsicles	BBQ Glazed Pork Chops	Vegan Pasta Primavera
22	Coconut Mango Rice Pudding	Lemon Garlic Herb Turkey Cutlets	Sweet Potato Black Bean Enchiladas
23	Berry Chia Seed Pudding	Moroccan Spiced Chicken	Vegan Lentil Sloppy Joes
24	Avocado Chocolate Mousse	Mushroom and Spinach Quesadillas	Lentil and Spinach Curry
25	Banana Chocolate Chip Muffins	Vegan Chickpea Curry	Moroccan Spiced Salmon

DAY	A	B	C
26	: Raspberry Coconut Popsicles	Chicken Caesar Salad	Vegan Cauliflower Curry
27	Lemon Blueberry Scones	Caprese Salad with Grilled Chicken	Vegan Ratatouille
28	Mango Coconut Rice Pudding	Black Bean and Corn Salad	Honey Lime Chicken Skewers
29	Strawberry Banana Parfait	Lentil and Vegetable Stir-Fry	Grilled Swordfish with Quinoa Salad
30	Apple Cinnamon Bread	Chickpea and Avocado Salad	Greek Lemon Chicken with Roasted Vegetables

Weekly Meal Planner

WEEKS	BREAKFAST	LUNCH	DINNER
MON			
TUE			
WED			
THU			
FRI			
SAT			
SUN			

Weekly Meal Planner

WEEKS	BREAKFAST	LUNCH	DINNER
MON			
TUE			
WED			
THU			
FRI			
SAT			
SUN			

Weekly Meal Planner

WEEKS	BREAKFAST	LUNCH	DINNER
MON			
TUE			
WED			
THU			
FRI			
SAT			
SUN			

Weekly Meal Planner

WEEKS	BREAKFAST	LUNCH	DINNER
MON			
TUE			
WED			
THU			
FRI			
SAT			
SUN			

Weekly Meal Planner

WEEKS	BREAKFAST	LUNCH	DINNER
MON			
TUE			
WED			
THU			
FRI			
SAT			
SUN			

Weekly Meal Planner

WEEKS	BREAKFAST	LUNCH	DINNER
MON			
TUE			
WED			
THU			
FRI			
SAT			
SUN			

Weekly Meal Planner

WEEKS	BREAKFAST	LUNCH	DINNER
MON			
TUE			
WED			
THU			
FRI			
SAT			
SUN			

Weekly Meal Planner

WEEKS	BREAKFAST	LUNCH	DINNER
MON			
TUE			
WED			
THU			
FRI			
SAT			
SUN			

NOTES

NOTES

NOTES

NOTES

NOTES

NOTES

NOTES

NOTES

NOTES

NOTES

NOTES

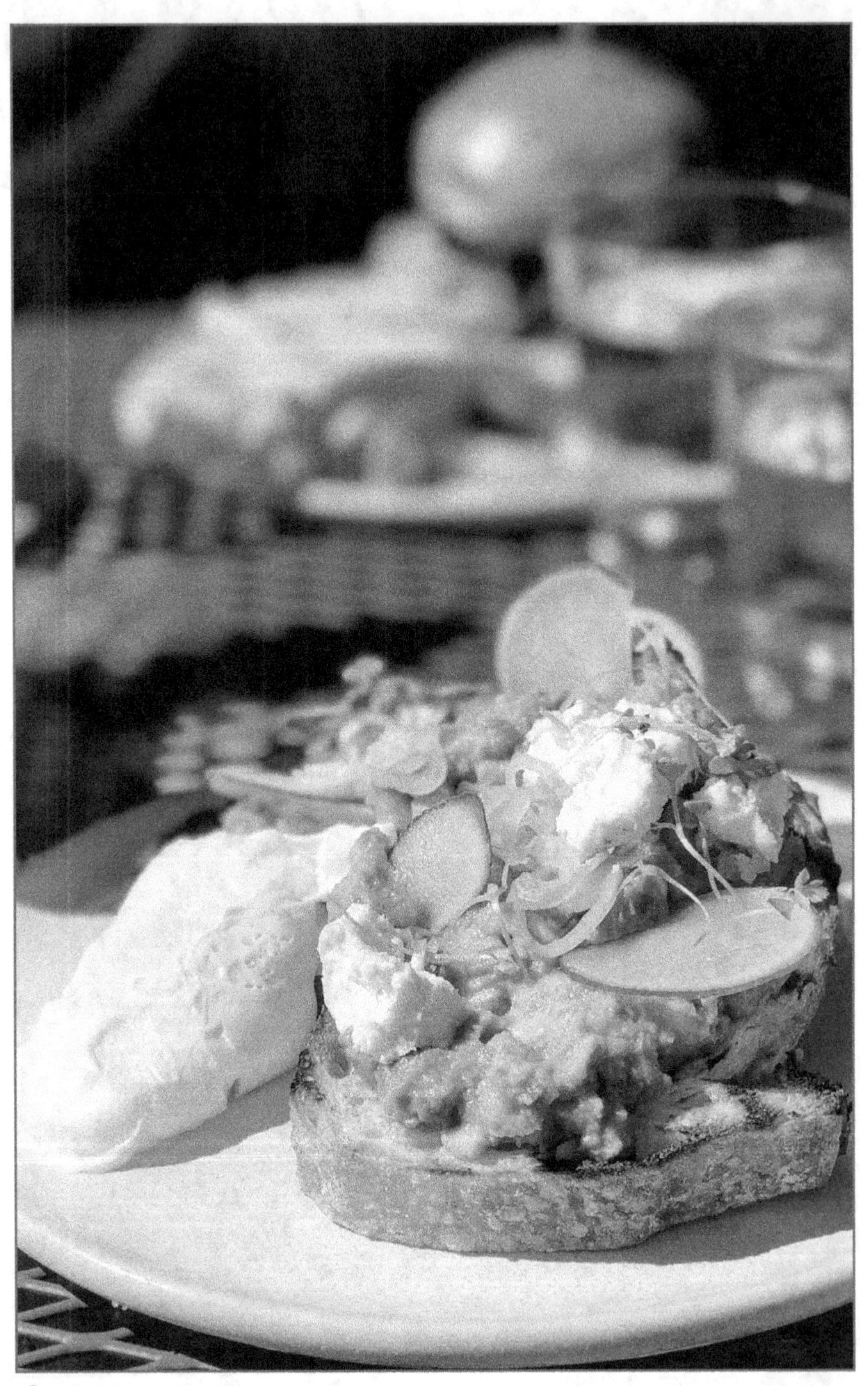